Conditioning Behavior & Psychiatry

Conditioning Behavior & Psychiatry

Thomas A. Ban

with a foreword by W. Horsley Gantt

AldineTransaction
A Division of Transaction Publishers
New Brunswick (U.S.A.) and London (U.K.)

First paperback printing 2008
Copyright © 1964 by Thomas A. Ban

This book is printed on acid-free paper that meets the American National Standard for Permanence of Paper for Printed Library Materials.

Library of Congress Catalog Number: 2008002627
ISBN: 978-0-202-36235-9
Printed in the United States of America

Library of Congress Cataloging-in-Publication Data

Ban, Thomas A.
    [Conditioning and psychiatry]
    Conditioning behavior and psychiatry / Thomas A. Ban.
        p. ; cm.
    Originally published: Conditioning and psychiatry. Chicago : Aldine, [c1964].
    Includes bibliographical references and index.
    ISBN 978-0-202-36235-9 (alk. paper)
        1. Conditioned response. 2. Psychiatry. I. Title.
    [DNLM: 1. Psychiatry—methods. 2. Behavior Therapy. 3. Conditioning (Psychology) WM 100 B212c 1964a]

BF319.B3 2008
153.1'526--dc22   2008002627

FOREWORD

SHAKESPEARE TO THE contrary—"the evil that men do lives after them, the good is oft interred with their bones"—many of the world's great thinkers have not attained to the eminence they deserved until long after their death. Some, like Mendel, William Blake, Gerald Manley Hopkins, Peirce (the creator of pragmatism), were scarcely recognized during their lives; others, whose talents are apparent in their day, become more famous later. Some whose greatness is admitted are always poorly understood; Emerson said that although Plato was appreciated through the ages as one of the greatest of men, there were often not more than a dozen alive at one time who understood him.

Pavlov falls partly into both of these groups, for his fame seems to be growing now 28 years since his death, but his concepts are still not clearly comprehended. Savich, one of Pavlov's collaborators, said to me in 1929 that he doubted whether more than six of Pavlov's students understood his book on conditional reflexes.

It is true that Pavlov's research on digestion was recognized by physiologists at the turn of the century (for this he won the Nobel Prize in 1903), and that the first impact of the conditional reflex was acclaimed by members of the school of behaviorists such as Watson. But the details of his work are still unknown today by most of those who write about him. Paradoxically, the excessive claims made by Watson for the conditional reflex have had a deleterious effect on the progress of Pavlovian concepts, similar to what has happened with Freudian ideas.

In the present decade there seems to be an awakening in

regard to the significance of Pavlov's teachings. Many people are concerned with the relation of Skinnerian operant conditioning to the "classical" Pavlovian type, but even with those whose efforts are in this field, there is little precise knowledge of the mass of data accumulated by the Pavlovian school. Especially is this true in the U.S.A.

To the small group of those who have conscientiously attempted to summarize and interpret the work emanating from Pavlov, it is a pleasure to welcome Doctor Ban. Ban is thoroughly acquainted with the work of Pavlov and his successors through his extensive reading as well as from personal experience of the application of these methods to the study of the human being. In performing this task of interpreting Pavlov and his followers, the author presents us with a scholarly treatise, tracing the historical development of the work from Locke to Sechenov to the major research of Pavlov, and including the contributions of the present decade.

Not only has Doctor Ban revealed himself as a scholar in this book, but he compliments the English language by having produced a monograph unusual in scientific writing for its clear and elegant phrasing—qualities rarely met with in our era of confused and hurried thinking and anxiety to get into print.

Ban has produced a book of great worth in the field of psychiatry. He has taken an important step toward placing the most confused of our medical departments on an objective basis. For the thoroughness of his comprehension and the excellence of his presentation of the work of Pavlov and his successors applied to psychiatry, I offer my gratitude and congratulations to Doctor Ban.

W. HORSLEY GANTT
The Pavlovian Laboratory
The Johns Hopkins University
and
Veterans Administration Hospital
Perry Point, Maryland

*Learn the ABC's of Science
before attempting to ascend
its heights. Never reach
for the next step before
having mastered the preceding
ones.*

PAVLOV

PREFACE

CONDITIONING IS one of the methods of psychiatry. It is a behavioral method, which has a stimulus-response constellation. The stimulus itself can be measured, changed, and combined, and the responses can be measured both qualitatively and quantitatively. The conditioning method utilizes the conditional reflex phenomenon. It is not a static situation, since, during the conditioning procedure, responses to certain stimuli are acquired where no responses existed previously. In more recent times behavioral conditioning expanded to include neurophysiological aspects and was correlated with psychic manifestations. To date there is no comprehensive work available that deals with the conditioning method, covering fully the behavioral, neurophysiological, and psychiatric aspects. This book is intended to fill that gap.

The purpose of the book is to describe the development of conditioning procedures since the introduction of the concept. It is primarily concerned with the analysis of elementary and complex behavioral observations, of neurophysiological and neuropathological discoveries as seen from the standpoint of psychiatric disorders. Since the book includes recent contributions to conditioning by other experimental methods and techniques (e.g., electrophysiological), the psychiatric view presented is, not purely the Pavlovian, but a modern approach to psychiatry stemming from a Pavlovian orientation.

Setting out as it does to provide a comprehensive view of the conditioning method, the book must be constructed in a systematic and detailed manner. It has been divided into five sections. In the first the conditional reflex phenomenon and the conditioning method are presented briefly in their historical perspective, taking the reader from the writings of Locke and Bentham through the discoveries of Bernard and of Bidder and Schmidt to the fundamental experiments of Pavlov. Then follows a résumé of the behavioral observations and methods of the Pavlovian school. This chapter is necessarily complemented by the interpretation of behavioral observations according to Pavlov's fuctional brain model. Part I is completed by a summary of present-day knowledge on the neurophysiology of conditioning.

Part II first sets out, in brief, the historical sequence in the correlation between psychopathology and pathological brain functions. Pavlov's concept of psychiatry as a clinical science is also touched upon. This leads to chapters on the Pavlovian concepts in general and clinical psychopathology. In Part III a description of the best-known conditioning techniques applied in human testing, particularly those which are applicable for diagnostic purposes, is discussed. Part III also includes a chapter on the test procedures elaborated by the use of these techniques and on the patterns that would be considered present in a normally functioning adult. Part IV is concerned with the clinical application of the method and discusses the findings and the implications that it has for psychopathology and therapy or, in general, for psychiatry. Part V contains a critical evaluation of the matter presented, followed by a bibliography and index.

It is perhaps superfluous to state that a book such as this could not have been written without considerable assistance. Many people assisted in preparing the book and to them all go my heartfelt thanks. It would be impossible to enumerate all those involved, but I wish to mention especially Dr. H. E. Lehmann, to whom a debt of profound gratitude is owed for the confidence he displayed in my ability to perform this task. From the very beginning he was a continuous source of help and encouragement. I am also indebted to Dr. W. H. Gantt, who through his translations and articles has been foremost in establishing in English the terminology of conditioning. Without his work the difficulty of preparing this book would have been greatly increased. I wish to express my gratitude to Mr. J. Kenyon for his conscientious editing of the first draft, to Mr. M. Donald and Mr. A. Jones for editing the second draft, and to Drs. H. Durost and V. Matthews who edited the final draft.

My sincere thanks go to Mrs. S. Schouten and Mrs. G. Teleky for their secretarial help in the preparation of the manuscript.

THOMAS BAN

CONTENTS

PART ONE

From Overt Behavior
to
Neurophysiology

INTRODUCTION
AND HISTORICAL
BACKGROUND

CONDITIONING IS a method that utilizes what has come to be known as the "conditional reflex phenomenon." The following definition is given in the *Oxford English Dictionary:* "Conditional: subject to, depending on, or limited by, one or more conditions, not absolute." For our purposes conditioning may be described as referring to the learning of some particular response. The conditional stimulus is one that was originally ineffective but that, after being paired with an unconditional stimulus, evokes the conditional response.

The first description of this phenomenon may be traced to an observation made in 1852 by Bidder and Schmidt. In the course of their experiments they discovered that teasing a dog with food led to gastric secretion. About the same time a similar observation was made by Claude Bernard. He noticed, while collecting gastric secretion from a horse, that after several repetitions the mere fact of his entering the stable provided sufficient stimulus to induce gastric secretion. Further observations of a similar kind were reported by Thorndike. All these phenomena remained a matter of mere academic interest until Pavlov together with Shoomova-Simanovskaya experimented with sham feeding of an esophagotomized dog in the early years of the twentieth century. The observation that mere sham feeding produced gastric secretion turned

Pavlov's interest to what he termed "psychic secretion." Assisted by Wolfson and Snarski, he began to investigate these phenomena. The term "psychic secretion" was to be replaced sometime later by the term "conditional reflex" secretion. The word "reflex" is defined as "involuntary action of muscle, gland, or other organ, caused by the excitation of a sensory nerve being transmitted to a nerve centre and thence 'reflected' along an efferent nerve to the organ in question" (*Oxford Dictionary*).

The process by which Pavlov deduced the term "conditional reflex" followed these lines. The occurrence of gastric secretion required direct stimulation (food); sham feeding of an esophagotomized dog also produced secretion, the secretion this time being obtained without actual stimulation of the stomach by food. Secretion was thus induced by the indirect stimulation of the stomach through the visual, olfactory, or gustatory characteristics of the food by the highest centers of nervous activity. This model was made the basis for his concept of "conditional reflex action."

The conditional reflex phenomenon had been known, but not referred to as such, before Pavlov's time. Bidder and Schmidt inferred a connection between behavior and cerebral activity from their observations of intact animals. Thorndike and his school (Yerkes, Watson, Parker, etc.) worked along the same lines, and their experiments constituted a major step forward. Perhaps the basic contribution made by Pavlov, and one which set the stage for further progress, was his adoption of the principle that in any experiment there should be only one variable, which could be measured against a controlled background. This basic principle had not been adhered to prior to Pavlov's time; never had one simple measurable behavioral function been isolated and then exposed alone to investigation. It becomes apparent then that Pavlov's success lay in his ability to reach a situation in which his experimental variable could be isolated. As Grey Walter expressed it: "His fame rests on his measurement of the responses to stimuli."

As the importance of this basic principle cannot be overemphasized, the procedure whereby it was observed and adopted is of primary interest. Pavlov's first experiments with his conditional reflex phenomenon were conducted under Botkin. At first, dogs were shown bread, and then they were given the bread to eat. This pattern was continued until *the presentation of bread alone* elicited salivation. Thus the presentation of bread could, after a while, elicit the same response as had previously been obtained by placing the bread in the dog's mouth. A visual signal replaced and elicited the same response as a gustatory signal. At this point Pavlov introduced artificially colored bread. This bread was then presented to the dog and elicited no salivary response whatsoever. At the same time, however, the dog continued to respond to the familiar visual signal (naturally colored bread), while remaining completely unresponsive to the unfamiliar visual signal (artificially colored bread). The basic part of the experiment was thus completed.

At this point Pavlov made a number of further observations. First, he saw that it was imperative to separate the animal from the investigator. Isolation of the animal was important, since any activity or movement might prove a disturbing factor. It was necessary to deprive the dog of all outside influences except the stimulus. This observation came about as a result of someone's entering the room during one of his experiments, a fact that caused the dog to be diverted, with the subsequent cessation of salivary secretion. Second, he saw that other artificial signals, differing in quality, such as a light or a bell, could be made to replace the presentation of bread. The procedure followed was exactly as before: a bell was rung, and the dog was given bread to eat. Salivation was elicited. After a number of repetitions the bell was rung but no bread was placed in the dog's mouth. As in the previous experiment, salivation was elicited by *the mere ringing of the bell.* This time, however, an entirely alien signal (a bell) was capable of eliciting salivary response.

About this time Pavlov devised a simple operation that would enable him to measure quantities of salivary secretion accurately. This operation consisted of exposing the internal end of the salivary duct by an opening in the dog's cheek. At the beginning of each experiment thereafter, Pavlov determined the amount of saliva elicited by a food stimulus (placing bread in the dog's mouth), such stimulus being adequate for salivary secretion. This he called the *unconditional stimulus.* Then he combined this unconditional stimulus with a neutral, or as he called it *conditional stimulus,* which initially did not elicit salivary secretion. The measurement of these conditional reflex responses and their developmental patterns and peculiarities formed the basis from which Pavlov generated his concept and interpretations of inferred brain mechanisms.

Other contemporary investigators were interested in the same phenomenon, although their descriptions and selections of systems were somewhat different. Pavlov concentrated primarily on the unconditional reflex food response and the unconditional reflex to acid. The reflex action in both these instances was salivary secretion. The unconditional reflex food response has already been described, and Pavlov elicited a similar response by placing acid in the dog's mouth. He believed the reflex to acid to be defensive by nature. Bekhterev had worked on another defensive reflex phenomenon, namely, the unconditional defensive reflex to painful irritation, which consisted of a withdrawal movement. His measurements were not clearly defined, however, since more than one variable was involved. He described the conditional reflex phenomenon as an "associative reflex." In Germany, Kalischer was concerned with motor activity. He called his conditioning method *die Dressurmethode* ("training method") and investigated the reflex food response, measuring the motor activity that is concomitant with secretion. The measurement of the response to stimulation that Kalischer used was difficult to calculate, being the degree of motor activity associated with salivation. Pavlov, however, worked out all the aspects and patterns of the conditional reflex phenomenon. He applied them and inferred a complete reflex theory, in which all human behavior may be seen as unconditional and conditional responses in varying patterns. As a result, preference was given eventually to Pavlov's terminology, which became accepted usage in conditioning studies. To Pavlov, conditioning was the beginning of a science and not a means to an end.

Pavlov's behavioral observations were extremely accurate

in their description, but his functional brain model and his hypothetical constructions were schematic in their form.

It is widely acknowledged today that the application of the conditioning method is a valuable contribution to the understanding of certain brain functions. The original method, however, has now been supplemented by electrophysiological approaches and provides a basis for correlating behavioral, neurophysiological, and electrophysiological responses. These two aspects of conditioning, the behavioral and the electrophysiological, form the basis of the discussion developed in Part I. The conditioning method, with the inclusion of the electrophysiological approach places the Pavlovian "system" in a modern frame of reference.

The nineteenth century was to prove a milestone in the history of mankind, for it was in the course of this century that humanity at last began to place more importance on its own capacity for inventiveness than on the services that nature could render it. The social, the economic, and the scientific worlds were progressing by giant strides in their separate but interdependent ways. Industrialization reached hitherto undreamed-of heights, and its economy needed and therefore produced machinery of increasing refinement. This refinement in machine production gave rise to new scientific techniques, which in turn led to further scientific discoveries. These revolutionary changes altered the structure of society and led to a change in perspective of man's role in the order of things. In viewing the new "dominant man" of the industrial age, philosophers began to see humanity as the powerful shaper of its own destiny.

Although the concept of evolution was ancient and well known, its first appearance in philosophy came about in this period (Goethe, Erasmus Darwin, Lamarck). An evolutionary hierarchism was postulated by Spencer, gained wider acceptance, and was finally adapted to the field of neurophysiology in the work of Jackson.

Two widely accepted and flourishing doctrines of the nineteenth century were Locke's doctrine of the infant mind as a *tabula rasa,* to be written on by later experience, and Hartley's association principle elaborated upon by Bentham. In both cases the revolt against classical systems of thought is apparent. The progress of the human mind, in Locke's view, was from nil (the *tabula rasa*) through every collected and stored experience, the sum of which provided man with his knowledge, incentive, and capabilities. The new wave of scientists, arising in the latter half of the nineteenth century, found these deterministic philosophical theories congenial, and it was a mere step to transfer a philosophical concept to the field of physiology. We shall return to Locke's philosophy later in discussing his influence on Sechenov. Bertrand Russell has declared that Bentham's doctrine embraces, in its essence, the Pavlovian theory of the conditional reflex. Pavlov's concepts, however, because of their physiological nature, gave rise to a physiological explanation of psychological phenomena, while Bentham's association of ideas, because of their philosophical basis, led to a psychology independent of physiology.

The major historical trend of philosophy, which has been briefly outlined, is to be found in the background of both the German and the French school of physiology. Both followed the new trend, which viewed man in a more deterministic fashion. Typical of the German school was Dubois-Reymond's assertion that all properties of living matter are subject to physical and chemical laws. He denied any notion of a mystical vital force supposedly working in biological systems (a position, however, from which he was to retreat sometime later). Not only basic scientists but also clinicians joined the new approach. Griesinger, for example, made the now-famous declaration that "mental diseases are somatic diseases: that is diseases of the brain." He also asserted that there are no differences between organic and functional disorders, that psychiatry and neuropathology are, not merely two closely related fields, but one field in which "one language should be spoken" and in which the same laws prevail.

Among the leaders of the French school was Claude Bernard, who believed in the possibility of the organism as an entity that could be completely understood. He asserted that all functions are interrelated in varying patterns, thus forming a total organism, counteracting and interacting with outside influences. He also believed in an internal synthesis, which was the central nervous system. Bernard's concept of nervous inhibition (introduced by Budge and Hoffman in 1843) greatly influenced Sechenov, whose main work was on the analytical investigation of neuronal inhibition. He conducted his experiments on the central nervous system of the frog, and in his monograph *Reflexes of the Brain,* elaborated the idea that all activity, including the psychological, is reflex and as such follows fixed laws determinable by investigation.

The particular aspect of the historical and philosophical streams that was to become the forerunner of the conditioning method is to be found in the rise of neurophysiology, the origins of which lie in the supposition that the brain is the central organ of the higher forms of activity. This view had been in existence but remained a hypothesis unsupported by evidence for many centuries. Its modern development can be traced to the introduction of the theory of reflex activity. Descartes published his reflex theory on the philosophical level, which led to the introduction of the term "reflex" into physiology by Prokhaska (1788). Prokhaska considered the reflex as "reflection of a sensation in action." The discovery of the importance of the reflex arc in the nervous system, however, came only with Magendie and Bell, when it was adopted into neurophysiology. Prior to the time of Magendie and Bell, only a few investigators, such as Whyte and Hales, had pointed to the importance of the spinal cord in reflex action. The main emphasis had hitherto been placed (by Pfleuger and others) on investigating the patterns of the reflex arc and the functional manifestations of the reflex act. Such investigators as Sherrington, Magnus, Beard, Ukhtomski, Orbeli, and others contributed immensely to our knowledge of the functions of the different parts of the central nervous system, built upon the basic notion of reflex activity. Their precise recording of phenomena, together with studies of the morphological substrata, contributed decisively to our knowledge of the reflex activity of the lower part of the central nervous system.

The turning point of the investigation of the physiological functions of the brain came in the seventies of the last century. Two new methods, stimulation and ablation, were introduced. In 1870 Fritsch and Hitzig demonstrated that electrical stimulation of certain cortical areas of a dog elicited movement of the contralateral extremity, while ablation of the same areas led to absence of, or disturbance of, motor functions. These experiments were later verified by Ferrier, Schafer, and Horsley. For the first time, experimental approach had demonstrated that the cortex is composed of "projective areas" that are the cortical counterparts of particular motor functions. The other areas of the cortex had not at this time been mapped out; their exact functions were unknown, and they were defined as "associative areas." The functional topography of the cerebral cortex having been described in this fashion, it was believed for many years that nothing further remained to be done in the field of reflex analysis. The neurophysiologist of that day, with the contemporary means at his disposal, could discern little in the nervous system of the consequences of previous experience apart from temporary alterations in the threshold.

The decisive and revolutionary contribution made by Pavlov altered and strengthened the whole approach. With his perfection of the scientific method of conditioning, it became apparent that the reflex concept had by no means been fully exploited, and a whole new road was opened leading to the systematic study of cerebral functions. The concept of the conditional reflex has from that time received the same emphasis, in regard to higher functions of the nervous system, as the concept of the spinal reflex has in regard to lower functions.

Pavlov's procedure in studying and applying the conditional reflex phenomenon can be outlined in three stages (Konorski). In the first stage the "foundations" of the conditional reflex were laid down, beginning with the circumstances necessary for the formation of the conditional reflex. At this point Pavlov made the important discovery that, besides the excitatory or positive reflex, there existed also an inhibitory or negative conditional reflex. The second stage consisted of studies carried out to determine the dynamics of the cortical processes and mutual interrelations of positive and negative conditional reflexes. Subsequently, the theory was formulated that cortical function represented a peculiar, continuously changing interplay of the excitatory and inhibitory processes. These were found to arise constantly in various parts of the cortex, extending and restricting each other in accordance with the ever changing external environmental conditional stimuli. In the third and final stage the phenomena of functional pathology were studied and related to typological problems.

The well-defined model, developed by Pavlov through these three stages, enabled him and his early followers to set out their findings in a systematic manner, to interpret them, and to lay the groundwork for further experiments. The purely neurophysiological nature of this model, based on the application of conditioning procedures, made possible a detailed and ordered notation of behavioral observations. These, then, in the hands of Pavlov's later followers, became the basis of a method of systematic physiological studies designed to describe the patterns of normal psychological activity and also their alterations or psychopathology.

BEHAVIORAL

OBSERVATIONS

THE PATHWAY TO the quantitative analysis of behavioral manifestations was opened by the research of Pavlov and his collaborators. The basic phenomenon that they investigated
intensively was the conditional reflex, conditioning being the
method devised to approach this problem. Pavlov's experiments
were conducted on dogs that had undergone a simple operation consisting of exposing the internal end of the salivary
duct through an opening made in the cheek. This operation
made possible an accurate measurement of the salivary secretion, either by counting the drops or by collecting them in a
graded container. The animal was isolated in order to exclude
any foreign, external stimulation, and the experimenter observed its behavior from an adjoining room, aided by mirrors.
The experiments conducted by Pavlov follow, in order of
sequence.

1. EXPERIMENT

A dog was fed by placing food in its mouth. Salivary
secretion was observed to start one or two seconds after feeding began.

Terminological Description. Food in close connection with
the sensory end organs of the oral cavity consistently elicits
salivary secretion. The food, therefore, is called an *unconditional stimulus* of alimentary salivation, and the resulting
salivary secretion is called an *unconditional reflex or response.*

The time interval between the beginning of the unconditional stimulus and the onset of the unconditional reflex is called the *latency time of the unconditional reflex* and is relatively short.

2. EXPERIMENT

Puppies, immediately following birth, were fed *only with milk*. The milk elicited salivation. After a while merely the sight of milk resulted in salivary secretion, this reaction taking place within five seconds. At this time the sight of bread or meat was ineffective in eliciting salivation in these puppies, although both stimuli resulted in salivation when placed in the puppies' mouths.

Terminological Description. The milk in contact with the sensory end organs of the mouth is an unconditional stimulus for salivary secretion, but, when the sight of the milk becomes a stimulus for secretion, it then becomes a visual *conditional stimulus* for salivation. The total action may be called a *conditional reflex*, implying that certain conditions (e.g., prior oral administration, etc.) are necessary for reflex development.

It was seen, for example, on a number of occasions in this experiment that the sight of milk preceded the feeding of milk before the conditional reflex was established. It was also seen that the unconditional stimulus (milk), a natural signal for salivary secretion through the gustatory end organs of the oral cavity, could be transformed into a conditional stimulus when it acted by means of another sensory organ—in this experiment, vision. The time interval between the start of the conditional stimulus and the start of the conditional reflex is called the *latency time of the conditional reflex* and is longer than that of the unconditional reflex.

3. EXPERIMENT

A metronome beat was made to precede feeding on a few consecutive occasions. After several such occasions, salivation began in response to the metronome alone, secretion starting nine seconds after the introduction of the metronome beat.

Terminological Description. The metronome beat is the conditional stimulus of the conditional reflex salivary secretion in this experiment. An artificial signal, previously neutral with regard to salivary secretion, thus is made to elicit secretion. The coincidence, or rather the consistent temporal relation, of the conditional and unconditional stimuli, in this order, may be termed an *association* and is the prerequisite for conditional reflex formation. The latency time is relatively long in this experiment, where the conditional stimulus is an artificial signal, being four to five times longer than the latency time of an unconditional reflex and about twice as long as that of the conditional reflex, in which the conditional stimulus is a natural signal.

Without a description of further similar experiments, it may be said that any previously indifferent exteroceptive or interoceptive stimulus may be used as a conditional stimulus.

4. EXPERIMENT

A conditional food reflex was established with the metronome beat, and then the length of the conditional stimulation was considerably increased. Salivary secretion first began immediately after an interval corresponding to the original termination of the conditional stimulus, but was later postponed to the end of the lengthened conditional stimulus.

Terminological Description. The postponement of the conditional reflex to the end of the prolonged conditional stimulation may be regarded as a retardation or delay, and the conditional reflex is called a *retarded or delayed reflex.* The period of delay or retardation may be regarded as an inactive phase and is contrasted with the terminal active phase.

5. EXPERIMENT

A metronome beat was presented—with a one-minute interval—before feeding. After several repetitions a conditional reflex was established, the reflex action occurring one minute after the conditional stimulus.

Terminological Description. The conditional reflex with a time interval between the conditional and the unconditional stimulus is called a *trace reflex*. When the time interval does not exceed one minute, one refers to *early trace reflexes;* if the interval exceeds one minute, one refers to *late trace reflexes.*

6. EXPERIMENT

Dogs were fed every thirty minutes. After several feeding periods, the dogs salivated spontaneously every thirty minutes.

Terminological Description. In this late trace reflex, the thirty-minute interval served as a conditional stimulus. When there is a reflex conditioned to time, it is referred to as *time conditioning.*

These six experiments, which form the basic models of the conditional reflex, dealt with interaction between two stimuli, the unconditional stimulus and the conditional stimulus (in differently programmed arrangements). These experiments provided a structural description of the basic conditional reflex patterns. Further experiments, in which the functional properties are discussed, follow.

7. EXPERIMENT

A metronome beat was combined with feeding. After the establishment of the conditional reflex, a new, stronger sound was introduced, following the conditional stimulus but preceding the conditional reflex. The dog turned in the direction of the new sound and did not respond to the conditional stimulus.

Terminological Description. In this experiment the new stimulus (a strong sound) produces a "startle" reaction, which temporarily interferes with the previously established conditional reflex. The "startle" reaction is called an *orienting reflex,* and the phenomenon observed by its action, *external inhibition.*

8. EXPERIMENT

A conditional food reflex was established with the metronome beat; thereafter the conditional stimulus was not associated with feeding. The conditional salivary secretion steadily decreased and eventually stopped.

Terminological Description. The association of the conditional stimulus with its unconditional stimulus, in a well-established conditional reflex, is called *reinforcement*. In failing to reinforce the conditional reflex, the conditional stimulus becomes ineffective. This is called *extinction* of the conditional reflex. It is the same as the transformation of a positive conditional stimulus and a positive conditional reflex into a negative one. The negative conditional stimulus does not result in action. Furthermore, the time for developing extinction is directly proportional to the frequency of non-reinforced conditional stimuli.

9. EXPERIMENT

A conditional reflex was established with the sight of food. After several presentations of food without feeding, the animal ceased to secrete saliva at the sight of food, but after forty-five minutes' rest conditional salivary secretion recurred spontaneously.

Terminological Description. This experiment showed a spontaneous reappearance of the conditional reflex after a certain length of resting time.

10. EXPERIMENT

A positive conditional food reflex was established with a metronome beat and the sight of a black rectangle. Thereafter, only the metronome beat was repeatedly used without reinforcement. Salivary secretion to the metronome beat decreased rapidly and finally stopped but remained unchanged upon presentation of the black rectangle.

Terminological Description. Repetition of one of the two positive stimuli without reinforcement results in a decrease of salivary secretion following presentation of this stimulus. This is the same type of *internal inhibition* formerly described as extinction. The transformation phenomenon from a *positive* to a *negative conditional stimulus* is due to non-reinforced repetition.

11. EXPERIMENT

A conditional food reflex was established with a metronome beat. After several unreinforced repetitions of the metronome beat, the animal stopped secreting saliva. Following the presentation of the metronome beat, a black rectangle was presented, resulting in salivary secretion and recurrence of the conditional reflex for a very limited length of time.

Terminological Description. The extinguished conditional reflex reappears upon presentation of another stimulus (in this case, presentation of the black rectangle after the metronome beat). The reappearance of the conditional reflex to the original conditional stimulus is limited with respect to time. It is a type of external inhibition, namely, to the effect that the new stimulus *inhibits the inhibition*. The phenomenon of a stimulus (in this experiment the black rectangle) interfering with extinction is called *disinhibition*. This phenomenon and the term apply not only to extinction but also to other types of inhibition.

12. EXPERIMENT

A conditional food reflex to a metronome beat was established. The presentation of a black rectangle was then combined with the metronome beat. The combined stimuli stopped conditional salivary secretion. (This experiment was performed by Zavadsky in Pavlov's laboratories.)

Terminological Description. In this experiment the conditional stimulus (metronome beat) of an established conditional reflex coincides with a previously indifferent stimulus (black rectangle). In the new combination the positive conditional stimulus loses its effect, and this also occurs if the previously indifferent stimulus precedes the conditional stimulus by a short time interval (within fifteen seconds). This phenomenon is called *conditional inhibition.*

13. EXPERIMENT

A conditional food reflex was established to a metronome beat of a certain frequency. Temporarily, salivary secretion was observed to develop to any other frequency of the metronome beat.

Terminological Description. Stimuli bearing some qualitative or quantitative resemblance to the conditional stimulus may temporarily result in a conditional reflex. This phenomenon may be called *generalization of the conditional stimulus.*

14. EXPERIMENT

A conditional food reflex was established and reinforced to a certain metronome frequency. Salivary secretion was obtained with other frequencies similar to the conditional stimulus. Initially, the amount of salivary secretion to the neighboring metronome frequencies was significantly less than to the reinforced conditional stimulus. Later, secretion to the non-reinforced neighboring frequencies increased continually until it reached the amount of salivary secretion obtained with the reinforced conditional stimulus. Thereafter it began to decrease and eventually ceased to develop altogether to the non-reinforced neighboring frequencies.

Terminological Description. In this experiment one can see the initial generalization of the conditional stimulus from a certain frequency to the neighboring frequencies. Later, the opposite phenomenon may be observed, namely *differentiation,* in which the conditional reflex again becomes limited to its original conditional stimulus, that is to say, none of the neighboring metronome beat frequencies elicits it any longer. This differentiation may be called *differential inhibition,* since the conditional stimulus inhibits all other stimuli in respect to conditional reflex formation.

15. EXPERIMENT

Mechanical stimuli were applied on four tissue areas of the skin above the heel. Positive conditional reflexes were established on the upper three by association and reinforcement with food, these conditional reflexes being equal in strength. Mechanical stimulation of the lowest area was never associated with food. After stimulation of this inhibitory area, the secretory effect of the previously equal positive reflexes was changed. Immediately after the stimulation of the inhibitory area, stimulation of the nearest positive point to this area did not result in any conditional salivary secretion. The stimulation of the second, previously positive area led to a marked fall in secretory effect. The salivary secretion was unchanged in the case of the upper area at this time. A short time later, the stimulation of the second area did not result in salivation any more, and the stimulation of the upper area led to a marked fall in secretory effect. Conditional salivary secretion to the stimulation of the upper area also decreased finally to nil with the lapse of time. However, at a later stage the positive conditional reflex was completely re-established at the upper point and later at the middle points and, finally, even on the point nearest to the area of application of the negative inhibitory stimulus. (This experiment was performed by Krasnogorski and Petrova in Pavlov's laboratories.)

Terminological Description. The negative or inhibitory effect is not static. In this experiment the negative conditional stimulus, applied to the lowest skin area, extended spatially. This phenomenon is called *irradiation.* Conversely, in the last stage of this experiment, when the effects of stimulation become "fixed" to the point of application, the phenomenon is called *concentration.* These terms may also be applied in cases of activity or excitation.

16. EXPERIMENT

A positive conditional food reflex was established to mechanical stimulation of the front legs, and a negative conditional reflex by stimulation to the hind legs. Areas beyond the locus of the positive conditional stimulus were stimulated, and the resulting salivary secretion approximated the amount obtained to the original positive conditional stimulus. Stimulation beyond the locus of the negative conditional stimulus did not result in any salivary secretion. The effects of stimulation vary between negative and positive areas; that nearer to the negative area resulted in decreased salivary secretion, and vice versa.

Terminological Description. According to this experiment, the effect of stimulation of areas around both negative and positive loci of the conditional reflex is determined by the sign of the locus. Between these areas the effect is determined by the relative strength of the opposing signs; for example, nearer to the negative area there is a decrease of salivary secretion to stimulation.

17. EXPERIMENT

A positive conditional food reflex was established to mechanical stimulation of the front legs. A similar stimulus was transformed into an inhibitory conditional stimulus of the hind legs by not reinforcing it. There was a significant increase in salivary secretion if the positive conditional stimulus of the front legs was administered immediately after the inhibitory stimulation of the hind legs.

Terminological Description. The phenomenon in which one process influences another consecutive process is called *induction.* In this experiment the first applied inhibitory or negative conditional stimulus has a positive influence on the secondarily applied excitatory or positive conditional stimulus. Since in this experiment the inhibitory process resulted in an increased salivary secretion of the positive conditional stimulus, the phenomenon is called *positive induction*. When the opposite effect is observed, that is, where the excitatory process results in an increased inhibition, the phenomenon is called *negative induction*.

18. EXPERIMENT

A positive conditional food reflex was established to mechanical stimulation of the front legs. A similar stimulation was transformed into an inhibitory conditional stimulus on the hind legs by not reinforcing it. The positive conditional stimulus was administered immediately after the inhibitory stimulus, and simultaneously an unpleasant substance was placed in the animal's mouth. No increase was observed in salivary secretion. (This experiment was performed by Fursikov in Pavlov's laboratories.)

Terminological Description. This experiment shows an effect similar to disinhibition and is achieved in this case by placing an unpleasant substance in the animal's mouth simultaneously with the conditional stimulus. This "disinhibitory-like" effect abolished the induction. Its effect is the inhibition of induction.

19. EXPERIMENT

Eight positive conditional food reflexes were established to mechanical stimulation of the skin in one line. Thereafter, one of these was extinguished. The inhibition irradiated in both directions (first phase). After the irradiation of inhibition reached its peak, leaving no positive areas of stimulation, concentration took place (second phase). At this stage there was a temporary increase in salivary secretion to mechanical stimulation in the neighboring consecutive spot of the last negative stimulation. Finally, the original situation was reestablished, consisting of one negative and seven positive conditional food reflexes. (This experiment was performed by Kogan in Pavlov's laboratories.)

Terminological Description. Irradiation and concentration

are in mutual interaction with the process of positive and negative induction. In this experiment the irradiation is followed by concentration. Thereafter, in the temporary increase of salivary secretion to mechanical stimulation in the neighboring consecutive spot of the last negative stimulation, one may recognize positive induction, induced by the initially irradiated and subsequently concentrated negative process.

20. EXPERIMENT

A conditional food reflex was established to a complex stimulus, consisting of two nearly identical metronome beats. The salivary secretions to the separate components were equal.

Terminological Description. With a complex stimulus, if its components are identical in intensity, the reflex responses to these components are also equal.

21. EXPERIMENT

A conditional food reflex was established to a complex stimulus, consisting of two metronome beats that were markedly different in intensity. The salivary secretion to the weaker beat, if administered alone, was zero.

Terminological Description. In a complex stimulus the stronger masks the weaker, and the weaker alone does not result in any reflex action. The full action is restricted to the effect of the stronger stimulus alone.

22. EXPERIMENT

A conditional food reflex was established to a complex stimulus consisting of two metronome beats that differed slightly in intensity. Thereafter, both stimuli were extinguished separately. The conditional reflex to the complex stimulus was not altered.

Terminological Description. This experiment is an example of the phenomenon of the *synthesis of stimuli* in a complex stimulus pattern. This synthesis in the complex stimulus is still effective in producing a conditional reflex, even after the individual components have been extinguished.

Experiments 7–22 discuss the functional characteristics of conditioning, for example, generalization, differentiation, positive-negative induction and their interaction. In all these experiments, however, there always existed a conditional reflex situation that might at times effect another conditional reflex situation. In the next experiment the "conditioning of the conditioning procedure" is described. This is the procedure used in the learning mechanisms of everyday life.

23. EXPERIMENT

The beat of a metronome was combined with feeding. After the establishment of the conditional reflex, a black rectangle was presented to the dog, preceding the metronome beat by fifteen seconds. When after several associations the conditional reflex developed to the black rectangle, mechanical stimulation was introduced fifteen seconds before the presentation of the black rectangle. After several associations, the conditional reflex developed in response to the mechanical stimulation. (This experiment was performed by Frolov and Fursikov in Pavlov's laboratories.)

Terminological Description. The conditional responses described in this experiment form a chain reflex *in toto*, and they are called primary, secondary, and tertiary conditional stimuli and conditional reflexes, with respect to their elements. In a chain reflex the conditional stimulus of a well-established conditional reflex serves as an unconditional stimulus of the consecutive conditional reflex in the chain—as, for example, the metronome beat for the rectangle, and the latter for the mechanical stimulation.

In the following experiments a number of the patterns of pathological alteration are described. These alterations have their basis in integrated defensive pathological patterns.

24. EXPERIMENT

Four conditional reflexes were established and administered consecutively, with an equal time interval and in the following order: metronome beat, the exhibition of a black rectangle, a tone stimulation, and a mechanical stimulation. The experiment was continued on the next consecutive day, but with a changed order of sequence. A decrease in salivary secretion was observed. (This experiment was performed by Soloveychik in Pavlov's laboratories.)

Terminological Description. In this experiment the sequences of positive conditional stimuli are integrated upon repetition. The result of this integration is called a *stereotype* and, since it is alterable, a *dynamic stereotype.* Changing the order of sequence in the dynamic stereotype (or, in general, interfering with or altering the integration) produces "strain," which results in inhibition, as is manifested by the decrease in salivary secretion.

25. EXPERIMENT

Conditional food reflexes were established to different positive and negative conditional stimuli. The conditional stimuli were presented day by day in the same order. Changing the sequence of the stimuli resulted in inhibition and a decrease in salivary secretion, and further change resulted in an increase in inhibition, which finally resulted in sleep.

Terminological Description. Changing the sequence of stimuli, or, in other words, the alteration of a dynamic stereotype, produces overstrain. This overstrain, or *ultramaximal stimulation,* results in an increasing inhibition, which finally induces sleep.

26. EXPERIMENT

A conditional food reflex was established to a particular frequency of a metronome beat. Other frequency metronome beats were differentiated from this. The difficulty of differentiation increased when the metronome beat frequencies came too close to each other. In parallel, salivary secretion decreased and eventually stopped. At this point the animal occasionally fell asleep.

Terminological Description. In this experiment the inhibition resulting from the overstrain of differentiation leads to a quantifiable decrease in the conditional reflex response and finally to cessation of salivary secretion and eventually to sleep.

The sleep here is seen as a special, more complex form of inhibition (internal) and is called *sleep inhibition.* This sleep inhibition is called *defensive,* or also *protective inhibition* by Pavlov, since it protects the central nervous system from the functional damage that may be caused by the overstrain.

27. EXPERIMENT

A conditional food reflex was established to a faint sound. The repetitive administration of this faint conditional stimulus resulted in a decrease of salivary secretion and an increase of inhibition, leading to sleep.

Terminological Description. The repetition of a weak conditional stimulus, without reinforcement, creates an increase of inhibition, which is manifested in a decrease of salivary secretion. The final result is sleep.

28. EXPERIMENT

Two grams of chloral hydrate were administered rectally to a dog. Thereafter, two positive conditional food reflexes of different strengths and a single negative conditional reflex were established. At the beginning of the chloral hydrate action, the amounts of saliva secreted to either of the positive stimuli were equal, but later there was a considerably larger amount of salivary secretion to the weaker stimulus than to the stronger. Finally, the negative conditional stimulus resulted in salivary secretion, whereas none followed the positive conditional stimulus. (This experiment was performed by Lebedinskaya in Pavlov's laboratories.)

Terminological Description. According to this experiment, sleep inhibition induced by chloral hydrate goes through different stages. The first stage is the so-called *equivalent stage,* the second the *paradoxical,* and the third the *ultraparadoxical.* The phenomena corresponding to these stages are equalization of salivary secretion to the different stimuli in the equivalent stage (quantitatively the same salivation to the stronger and weaker conditional stimuli), greater effect to the weaker and less effect to the stronger stimulus in the paradoxical stage, and a positive response to the negative stimulus and a negative response to the positive stimulus in the ultraparadoxical stage.

The following group of experiments describes what happens when the defensive inhibition breaks down and pathological behavior results.

29. EXPERIMENT

A positive conditional food reflex was established to the projection of a circle, and a negative conditional food reflex to the projection of an ellipse. Differential inhibition was easily established when the ratio of the circle to the ellipse was 2:1. The proportion was gradually altered during the experiment, toward the ratio 9:9, but the animal was unable to differentiate between the circle and the ellipse even when the ratio was 9:8. At this stage the dog became increasingly nervous and excited, and its previously established differentiations were also affected. After the dog had had considerable rest, the 2:1 differentiation was again established. Upon repetition of the experiment, the dog broke down again at the 9:8 ratio. (This experiment was performed by Shenger-Krestovnikova in Pavlov's laboratories.)

Terminological Description. Beyond certain limits of the ability to discriminate—for example, the 9:8 ratio in this experiment—an animal fails to differentiate. This failure is accompanied by increasing nervousness and excitation. The increasing nervousness and excitation is called *experimental neurosis,* since it bears a resemblance to the neurotic condition in humans, and is experimentally induced.

30. EXPERIMENT

Conditional food reflexes were established with two dogs. The positive conditional stimuli were a metronome beat, mechanical stimulation of the hind legs, and the sound of a bell. The negative conditional stimuli were mechanical stimulation of the forelegs and a whistle-metronome beat combination. In one of the experimental sessions, the hind and forelegs were simultaneously stimulated. The animals showed two different independent patterns of response to this alteration. In one dog the simultaneous administration of positive and negative conditional stimuli was followed by impairment of inhibitory functions, at first of retardation, then of conditional inhibition, and later of differential inhibition. In the other animal, the administration of positive and negative conditional stimuli was followed by impairment of the excitatory function, manifested in impaired positive conditional reflex formation.

Terminological Description. This experiment demonstrates that collision between the positive and negative conditional stimuli results in an impairment of performance. There are, however, different reactions to the collision; in one case we have excitation, and in the other, inhibition. On this basis one may differentiate between a so-called *strong or excitatory animal* and a so-called *weak or inhibitory animal.* In the strong type, the collision results in an extreme state of excitation as a result of the decomposition of the processes of inhibition, at first of retardation, then of conditional inhibition, and finally also of differentiation. In the weak type, the overstrain results in an extreme inhibition as a result of the decomposition of the processes of excitation, shown in the effect of the positive conditional reflex, which diminishes and finally ceases.

31. EXPERIMENT

Conditional food reflexes were established. One of the dogs belonged to the strong and one to the weak type. A positive conditional reflex was established to a metronome beat of 120/min, and a negative conditional reflex to a metronome beat of 60/min. Immediately after, the negative conditional stimulus was continuously reinforced with feeding in both dogs, in an attempt to change the negative conditional stimulus into a positive conditional stimulus, and the positive conditional stimulus was no longer reinforced. This was comparatively successful in the animal of the strong type. In the weak type the effects of the two metronomes remained isolated and were not transformable into one another; furthermore, they showed a high degree of stability.

Terminological Description. The basis of the phenomenon of changing a positive conditional stimulus into a negative and a negative conditional stimulus into a positive is *mobility*. Such a phenomenon was presented in this experiment by the dog of the strong type. The absence of mobility is called *inertia*. Inertia was presented in a high degree, or as a "pernicious" type of stability of the conditional stimuli, by the dog of the weak type.

Pavlov summarized these experiments in his twenty-three lectures presented at the Russian Military Academy in 1924. The first edition of the material was published in 1926, the second in 1927, and the third in 1935. The schematic outline of the experiments follows the general order of Pavlov's presentation, but details of the precise quantification of the experiments are omitted in this description.

The foregoing experiments have described in brief the structural characteristics of the conditional reflex, together with the functional patterns, their dynamics and breakdown. It should be pointed out that this is an attempt to describe psychological functioning in its entirety through measurable behavioral manifestations.

In his lectures Pavlov offered an interpretation of be-havioral observations in terms of inferred brain processes. On the basis of the cortical representation of the visceral organs and of the somatic areas, Pavlov maintained that cortical activity, in its interaction with the external world, is projected into behavior and, conversely, that behavior is projected in a representative way onto the cortex. He also stressed that the energy for the cortical activity of the brain arises from sub-cortical centers.

The terminology introduced after each of the experiments described above was that created by Pavlov to handle the observed behavioral phenomena. The following chapter will demonstrate how this same terminology was employed in dis-cussing his brain model.

PAVLOV'S BRAIN MODEL

AND CONCEPTS

THE ANTECEDENTS OF Pavlov's brain model may be traced directly to the concepts of Sechenov and Jackson, who were both pioneers in the field of neurophysiology. Sechenov and Jackson, in their turn, were influenced by the philosophical concepts of Locke and Spencer, respectively. Locke promulgated the theory that psychological development of the mind depends entirely on the activity of the sense organs, a theory expressed in his famous doctrine that the mind of a newborn child is a *tabula rasa,* which is written on by experience alone. Sechenov, with his reflex theory, elaborated on Locke in his monograph *Reflexes of the Brain* (1863). According to Sechenov, all acts of life, both physical and psychological, are basically reflex, and any voluntary, involuntary, or psychological action in the reflex arc begins with a sensory stimulus-impulse related excitation and continues by means of a definite psychophysical act ending in muscular activity. In this view, not only psychological development, but all activity, depends entirely on the activity of the sense organs.

Jackson repostulated Spencer's evolutional hierarchism and adapted it to physiology. In Jackson's view, the lowest level consists of centers extending from the tuber cinereum to the conus medullaris, which he called "representative centers," since each center represents only a limited region of the body. The second level, of "re-representative centers," consists of the cortical voluntary motor centers and possibly the corpus striatum, in which wider regions of the body are incorporated.

The third and highest level, which includes the prefrontal and orbital lobes, is the most complex and least organized and represents the widest regions of the body.

The concepts of Sechenov and Jackson have been incorporated in Pavlov's brain model, according to which the adaptation of the organism to its surroundings, on the first level, is a subcortical function and is accomplished by the unconditional reflexes. These unconditional reflexes being limited in scope, there is a similarly limited and crude adaptation to the environment on this level.

In Pavlov's view, adaptation of the organism to the environment is accomplished on the second level by cerebral hemispheric function, with the exception of the frontal lobes. At this level, a new principle of activity is introduced by means of conditional connections. The new system is the signaling of external agents by numerous other so-called conditional agents, thus promoting an extremely varied orientation and adaptation to the environment. According to Pavlov, this constitutes the unified first-signal system of the organism. Another system of signaling is added at the third level by the introduction of the frontal lobes. By means of this new system, the signals of the first system may be resignaled. This new system is speech.

Speech, the third level, introduces a new principle of higher activity, making possible abstraction and generalization of the multitude of first-system signals. In consequence, it permits limitless conditioning and finely regulated adaptation to the surrounding world. To Pavlov this second system of signaling is the highest attainment in evolution and is a special human characteristic. Although all three levels of evolution are represented in Pavlov's model, the Pavlovian school's main achievement remained concentrated for a long time at the middle level, where it dealt with the patterns of the first-signal system.

Even after Pavlov's "excursion" into psychiatry, the orientation of his school continued to be toward his classical conditioning method, and the application of verbal, secondary system signals did not bring about any significant alteration in this scheme. However, the idea of investigating all normal and pathological phenomena by means of this method and describing them in Pavlov's terms seemed full of promise. He also thought that the basic patterns of functioning of the first- and second-signal systems were similar.

Pavlov's model, therefore, is based on the assumption that all nervous activity is reflex and, as such, a reaction to the stimuli of the external or the internal world (Locke and Sechenov), effected through the nervous system.

All reflex activity, according to Pavlov, has one of two forms: unconditional or conditional, and the entire reflex arc of any reflex consists of three main parts: afferent, central, and efferent. The afferent, or first part, includes that section stretching from the peripheral sensory end organ of the centripetal nerve to the sensory areas of the central nervous system. This section of the reflex arc, because it breaks down the entire world into stimulating units, is called an "analyzer," and the higher the animal in the phylogenetic scale, the more refined the analysis.

The second or central part of the reflex arc is the so-called coupling, connecting, or locking apparatus of the central nervous system, through which the central end of the analyzer is connected to the third part of the reflex arc. This efferent part determines the adaptive response.

That group of reflexes which is congenital is called "unconditional." Members of the other group are called "conditional," since their existence depends upon a continuous formation process through the life of the individual. They depend upon a multitude of external and internal conditions and upon the connective capacity of the central nervous system and are, therefore, constantly fluctuating in response to changing circumstances.

At the basis of any conditional reflex lies an unconditional reflex. The stimulation via signals, which bear no relationship to the unconditional response, is always built upon the initial stimulation of an unconditional reflex, provoked by the adequate unconditional attributes of an object. Pavlov assumed from this that the points of the central nervous system, which are strongly stimulated during the unconditional reflex, attract the weaker conditional stimulus impulses arising simultaneously from the external or internal environment. This is his explanation of the formation of the brain paths that constitute conditional reflex formation.

This assumption was extended later in such a manner that those points of the central nervous system which are strongly stimulated simultaneously with the discharge of a conditional reflex might become the basis of secondary conditional reflexes and so on, comprising "chain reflexes."

The fundamental condition, therefore, necessary for the formation of the conditional reflex is that a stimulus entering the central nervous system must coincide with the strong stimulation of an unconditional reflex. Under these circumstances, the relatively weak impulse of the conditional stimulus produces a process of excitation that promotes the closing of the brain path to the effector part of the unconditional reflex, which constitutes conditional reflex formation. Under circumstances in which the conditional stimulus acts alone and the effector part of the unconditional reflex is absent, a conditional reflex cannot be formed and the conditional stimulus engenders in the brain a process of inhibition, which tends to cause conditional reflex dissolution.

The two elementary basic processes of the brain—namely, excitation and inhibition—have a tendency to spread. The central nervous system is steadily bombarded by a multitude of impulses, resulting in a constant stream of excitatory and inhibitory central processes. These processes interrelate, limiting and confining each other to definite areas, and produce corresponding fields of interaction on the surface of the cerebral cortex. The process of inhibition is much less stable than that of excitation, since under the influence of extraneous stimuli it is more easily and quickly suppressed, which led Pavlov to the assumption that the inhibitory process is on a higher level of evolution than is the excitatory.

Whereas excitation is unique, there are three separate forms of inhibition: external, internal, and sleep. External inhibition is a concept previously applied to the physiology of the spinal cord. It is said to occur when an external stimulus elicits nervous activity, which temporarily interferes with previously established conditional reflexes. The reason for this, according to Pavlov, is that, under the influence of the new focus of excitation in the cortex, the excitability of the points corresponding with other conditional reflexes is decreased.

Internal inhibition has several forms: extinction, differential inhibition, retardation (i.e., delay), and conditional inhibition. It develops as a consequence of certan particular relations between the conditional and unconditional stimuli that interfere with the process by which the conditional reflex is elaborated.

Sleep is a separate form of inhibition. It appears in the form of normal sleep through the different stages of hypnotic states. During sleep the activity of the higher part of the nervous system is "weaker." According to Pavlov, it may "functionally disappear" altogether. In this state there is no conditional reflex formation.

In summary, excitation invariably accompanies the varied activities of the animal during the waking stage. Inhibition may be seen in the role of "guardian" of the most reactive parts, defending from injury the central nervous system. Thus, during the time of optimal excitability, new conditional reflexes are easily formed, in contrast to the time when there is inhibition.

In Pavlov's model these basic processes have several patterns, hypothetically introjected from overt behavioral observations into the brain. These patterns are as follows:

1. *The pattern of closing of nervous paths (association), or conditional reflex formation:* Every strongly excited center (unconditional stimulus center) or strong excitation in some manner attracts toward itself energy from other weakly excited centers (conditional stimulus centers).

2. *The pattern of irradiation and concentration of nervous processes:* The processes of excitation and inhibition, originating from definite points of the cortex, under the influence of corresponding stimuli, irradiate over a larger area on the cortex prior to becoming concentrated in a limited space.

3. *The pattern of reciprocal induction:* Mutual induction

of the opposite process occurs. Pavlov maintained that when a stimulus destroys a given equilibrium in the cortex it passes over, wavelike, to the opposite process, the excitatory wave inducing an inhibitory wave, the inhibitory an excitatory.

4. *The pattern of the limit of the intensity of stimulation:* There is a maximum of non-injurious stress, beyond which inhibition, instead of excitation, always occurs. Beyond this point a strong stimulus may produce an equal or even weaker effect than a weak one.

5. *The pattern of the transition of the cortical cells into a state of inhibition:* If a positive conditional stimulus is unaccompanied by its unconditional stimulus for a certain length of time, the cortical cell, corresponding to this stimulus, then passes into a state of inhibition. The stimulus that conditions a process of inhibition in the cortex thus becomes a conditional, inhibitory, negative stimulus.

The activity of the cerebral hemispheres, according to Pavlov's model, is based on these five patterns. In addition, there are the functions of generalization, differentiation, and secondary conditional reflex formation, which are of the utmost importance in human development. Pavlov therefore regarded the cerebral hemispheres as presenting a "grandiose mosaic." Any external or internal stimulation is immediately represented on this mosaic as an excitation that, in accordance with the patterns of irradiation and concentration and of the mutual induction of the opposite process, produces a new equilibrium in the cerebral hemispheres. Since they are constantly receiving new stimuli, the cerebral hemispheres constitute, at any given moment, a system in a state of "dynamic equilibrium."

The pattern of the limit of the intensity of the stimulation is represented in Pavlov's brain model in the following manner. The intensity of the conditional reflex depends, within certain limits, upon the intensity of the conditional stimulus. (He referred to Gantt's demonstration that it also depends on the intensity of the unconditional stimulus.)

Beyond some maximum intensity of the conditional stimulus, however, variations in the effect may lead to three different

phases: equivalent, paradoxical, and ultraparadoxical. Such
conditional stimuli, which are too strong to produce a maximal
conditional reflex, were described by Pavlov as "transmarginal"
or "supermaximal" ("ultramaximal" in Gantt's English transla-
tion). In Pavlov's model, this inhibition is viewed as a protective mechanism by means of which the weak cortical cells
are protected from excessive excitation. The strength of the
stimulus necessary to produce paradoxical or pathological
changes varies in Pavlov's model and depends on the actual
equilibrium and the type of nervous system (temperament).

In this respect, Pavlov classified the nervous system in
accordance with three criteria: the force of the main nervous
processes, the degree of their mutual equilibrium, and their
mobility. According to this classification, the temperament of
the animal can be strong or weak (manifested in the basic
processes), balanced or unbalanced (of the excitatory and
the inhibitory process), and mobile or inert (changeable or
rigid basic processes). Excitation predominates in "choleric"
and "sanguine" animals, inhibition in those which are "phlegmatic" and "melancholic." All these types obviously correspond
to Hippocrates' classification. The choleric type corresponds to
Pavlov's strong but unbalanced type, which has strong excitatory and inhibitory processes, but with the excitatory process
predominating. The melancholic is generally represented by
the weak type in Pavlov's model, while the sanguine type
corresponds with his strong and well-balanced type. The
phlegmatic type corresponds to the strong, well-balanced, but
inert animal.

The extreme groups, choleric and melancholic, are liable
to break down in such a way that the choleric loses its
capacity for inhibition, while the melancholic shows a weakening of excitation. Pavlov emphasized, however, that, beyond a
tolerable stress, sanguine and phlegmatic animals also break
down.

Pavlov's brain model included further functional characteristics. According to the pattern of negative induction, cortical
excitation exerts an inhibitory action upon the subcortical
centers. Through this inhibitory action of the cortex the sub-

cortical centers can maintain a dynamic equilibrium, which is the proper relationship between the organism and the environment. (Here it should be noted that on several occasions Pavlov expressed his belief that the active state of the cortex is continually maintained by stimuli, arising from these subcortical centers.)

Analyzing and synthesizing functions are also included as functions of the cerebral hemispheres in Pavlov's brain model. By "analysis" is meant the decomposition of the whole into parts; by "synthesis" is meant the gradual reconstruction of the whole from its units or elements. The cerebral hemispheres carry out a thorough analysis and synthesis of the external and internal milieu, either differentiating or combining their separate elements. The external and internal conditions, through this analysis, become numberless signals.

Analysis, differentiating the positive conditioning signals from those which are inhibitory or negative, is based upon the process of *reciprocal induction,* while synthesis is accomplished by the process of conditional connections. The basis of analysis is provided by the peripheral endings of all the afferent nerve conductors, each being specially adapted for transforming a definite kind of energy into the general process of stimulation. As a rule, this stimulation-produced impulse, upon reaching the cerebral hemispheres, diffuses or irradiates, and synthesis follows. This is completed, to use Pavlov's term, by a "switching-on" of these nerve currents that lead to aggregate formation.

The two processes of irradiation and "switching-on" occur simultaneously. Irradiation, however, is gradually limited, and the excitation becomes concentrated, its limitation being effected by the other essential nervous process of inhibition. The inhibitory process irradiates in a manner similar to the excitatory process, and finally it too becomes concentrated. Analysis begins with the special work of the peripheral apparatus of the afferent conductors and is completed in the cerebral hemispheres by the inhibitory process. This physiological activity is continuous and simultaneous in the central nervous system.

The activity of the nervous system in the model is directed toward unification, integrating the work of all the parts of the organism, and also toward connecting the organism with the surrounding milieu, and, furthermore, toward establishing an equilibrium between the systems of the organism and external conditions. Pavlov divided nervous activity of behavior into lower and higher divisions, the former referring solely to connecting and the latter to integrating activity as well.

The principal manifestations of behavior are seen in muscular activity, accompanied to some extent by secretion due to the activity of glandular tissues. The muscular movement, beginning at the lower level with the activity of separate muscles and small groups of muscles, reaches a higher integration in the form of locomotor acts. In addition, the organism performs special movements in accordance with the principles of the preservation of the organism and of its species. These Pavlov termed unconditional, special, or complex reflexes, also called instincts, tendencies, or inclinations. Among them he furthermore distinguished organism or individual and species reflexes according to their function. The anatomical substrata of these activities supposedly lie in the subcortical centers, for example, in the basal ganglia.

These unconditional reflexes constitute the basis of the external behavior of the animal, upon which the conditional reflexes are developed to become the complete behavior.

We have presented Pavlov's brain model briefly in this chapter. The full description, covering his twenty years of objective study of the higher nervous activity of animals may be found in the first volume of his *Lectures on Conditioned Reflexes,* edited and translated by W. H. Gantt.

4

THE NEUROPHYSIOLOGICAL BASIS OF CONDITIONING

WITH THE PASSAGE of time Pavlov's method has become more and more influential in the field of physiological psychology and his terminology has found even greater application. A survey of Pavlovian classical conditioning would be incomplete without mentioning the relevant neurophysiological observations that have arisen in recent research.

The first stage of research in this area was to retest Pavlov's basic hypothesis on the role played by the cerebral cortex. This was followed by an attempt to determine the role of the various cerebral structures in conditional reflex formation and to establish the electroencephalographic correlates of conditional responses.

ROLE OF THE CEREBRAL CORTEX IN CONDITIONING

Experimental studies since the 1930's have shown that, contrary to Pavlov's belief, the cerebral cortex is not essential for conditioning. However, as Hilgard and Marquis pointed out, its importance does increase throughout the phylogenetic scale. Koller and Mettler demonstrated that, although reflexes can be formed in decorticated animals as rapidly as in normal animals, the former show no refinement in their conditional reflexes with practice. Conditioning, therefore, can take place in subcortical structures, but, as demonstrated, practice does not lead to refinement in this instance.

Pavlov's original hypothesis on the role of the cerebral cortex, which had for many years been lying in abeyance, was dramatically revived when Popov (1948) found that a conditional sound stimulus associated with electrical shock produces changes traceable on the electroencephalogram. The observed changes disappeared under ether narcosis, and Popov thought that they were of cortical origin without simultaneous changes in the subcortical areas. This led Popov to confirm the Pavlovian hypothesis that the conditional reflex is a cerebral cortical function and further led to renewed discussions in this area of research.

Sager and his associates restated the formerly held observation that after complete decortication of the animal the conditional reflexes are not totally abolished. Although the classical defensive conditional reflex can no longer be elicited after complete removal of the cerebral cortex, decorticated animals do show a vegetative and affective conditional reaction, which is more easily extinguished than the classical conditional reflex. A similar view was held by Hernandez-Peon. Bromiley found that, after the removal of the neocortex, a crude type of differentiation still remained as long as the upper brain stem and rhinencephalon were intact. This was further elaborated by Kupalov, who found that cats, after removal of their neocortex, can be conditioned to find food in a maze and differentiate between metronome frequencies and flicker or steady light, but after removal of their archipallium they lose the latter abilities. Decorticated animals also lose their delayed reflexes. Furthermore, it was established that partial mutilation of the cortex does not affect conditioning (except for modifications, i.e, differentiation, delayed reflex formation, etc.), and, even when the supposed cortical conditional and unconditional analyzers are divided by section, conditioning usually remains intact.

These experiments clearly showed that Pavlov's classical hypothesis regarding the monopoly the cortex held as the anatomical location of conditional reflex formation was no longer tenable.

ROLE OF VARIOUS STRUCTURES IN CONDITIONAL REFLEX FORMATION

Pavlov thought of conditioning in terms of the spread of fields of cortical excitation and inhibition. Shortly afterward, however, Konorski surmised a potential connection between emitting (or conditional) and receiving (or unconditional) centers. This conception was replaced by the assumption that a punctiform closure was at the basis of conditional reflex formation (Eccles, Gastaut). The latter was no longer based on inferences from behaviorally observed manifestations but was engendered by new methods, that is, electrophysiological instrumentation, implanted electrodes, microelectrode techniques, multichannel toposcope (Livanov), etc.

At first the technique of achieving conditional reflexes by direct brain stimulation, and therefore the proof of the non-necessity of the peripheral afferent pathways in conditional reflex formation, was developed. Gantt and his associates, by pairing a conditional auditory stimulus with unconditional direct cerebellar stimulation, were able to elicit, after repeated combination of the stimuli, the cerebellar response to the auditory signal alone. He obtained similar findings by placing the electrodes that provided the unconditional stimulus on the dorsal nerve roots of the spinal column. Further confirmation was received by Lilly, who placed his electrodes, providing the unconditional stimulus, in the center of the cerebellum, and by Rusinov, who applied direct current to the motor cortex of the rabbit as unconditional stimulus. More recently, conditioning has been achieved by the direct application, not merely of the unconditional stimulus, but of both conditional stimulus and unconditional stimulus. Guirgea, stimulating the visual cortex (conditional stimulus) and then applying an unconditional stimulus to the motor cortex, found that after several associations (roughly twenty) stimulation of the visual cortex alone resulted in the motor response.

After the non-necessity of afferent peripheral pathways in conditioned reflex formation had been established, the proof of the non-necessity of the peripheral efferent pathways in conditional reflex formation was developed by the utilization of central electrical (EEG registration) rather than behavioral responses. Loomis, Harvey, and Hobart (1936) observed that a previously indifferent tone, if presented with an unconditional light stimulus several times in succession, "blocked" the occipital alpha rhythm of the brain, taking on the role of the unconditional stimulus. They also noted that this alpha block response to the tone was extinguishable by withholding the reinforcement (light stimulus). The assumption that the efferent peripheral pathways were not essential for conditional reflex formation was further supported by Knott and Henry (1941), Jasper and Shagass (1941), and others.

The continuous improvement in instrumentation and the knowledge gained from this information pointed to an increasingly complex role of conditioning for the central nervous system.

The problem of the role of the different cerebral structures in conditioning was brought into a new frame of reference by three great discoveries. Magoun showed that local stimulation of the midbrain reticular formation desynchronizes the cerebral rhythms that accompany an increased cortical activity, while depression of the same structures enhances cerebral synchrony and reduces cortical activity. Jasper showed that stimulation or depression of the thalamic reticular formation has the same action, but only upon the region corresponding to the locus of stimulation, and Eccles assumed the presence of convergence of stimuli in the brain reticular structures.

Integrating these findings, Gastaut's school summarized the hypothetical role of different morphological structures in the conditioning procedure. According to them, the application of a stimulus at the beginning of any conditioning procedure results in a startle response with its visceral effects and generalized desynchronization of the electroencephalogram. This corresponds with the activation of the brain stem reticular formation. The startle response is followed by a reaction of attention. (orientating response), in which Gastaut pointed out the additional influence of the intralaminar and thalamic reticular nuclei with their more localized desynchronization of electroencephalographic activity. Thus Gastaut contrasted the primitive—undifferentiated signal—emotional quality of the startle response to more appropriately attentive recognition in the orienting reflex. During conditioning, after repetitive combination of two stimuli, the formerly indifferent conditional stimulus, when conditioned, evokes desynchronization of the electrical activity of the corresponding region of the unconditional stimulus, thus supposedly involving an infracortical closure between the afferent pathways of the conditional and unconditional stimuli. The closure is accompanied by the activation of the corresponding thalamocortical segment, resulting in the desynchronization of the electrical activity in the cortical field responsible for the behavioral reaction. He further supported these findings with evoked potentials traced by special electroencephalographic techniques. The primary evoked potential is produced by the unconditional stimulus and is due to the manifestation of specific afferentation of the midbrain reticular systems. The *conditioned* stimulus produces not a primary, but a secondary, evoked potential in the region of the unconditional stimulus. The closure, which makes this possible, is the result of "the convergence of heterogenous sensations on the neurons, involved in the closure." As a consequence of the closure, caudal projections are carried by the motor neurons and by preganglionic neurons of the vegetative system, while rostral projections are manifested in secondary evoked potentials in the analyzer areas of the unconditional and conditional stimuli. With these findings as a basis, Gastaut assumed that the site of the closure is in the brain stem (Brazier).

The role of the brain stem reticular formation in the formation of the conditional reflex has been described, and, although it has not been generally accepted as the "site of the closure," its important facilitating effect on conditional reflex formation was supported by Bremer, Bell, and others. Magoun supplemented the classical view of Pavlov on conditional reflex formation (functional links between the cortical areas of different analyzers), describing the modification of activity produced in the brain by the influence of reinforcing mechanisms in the brain stem. A similar view was presented by

Kreindler and Chang. Kreindler emphasized that the reticular formation may play a role in retention of traces (memory) as a storage without which conditional reflex formation would be impossible, but he also emphasized the fact that, while delayed reflexes were impaired, a mesencephalic lesion failed to abolish the conditional reflex. The reticular formation of the brain stem, according to Kreindler, seems to have the role of increasing the non-specific capacity of the prosencephalic neurons. Thus he assumed that the temporary connection is elaborated at a supramesencephalic level. Brain stem reticular stimulation increases the rapidity of the elaboration of the conditional reflex and conditional stimulus differentiation. His finding that a reticular fit greatly facilitates conditional reflex formation supported this view. Chang concluded the same by following a different experimental design and instrumentation. By using microelectrodes, probing microstructures, he found that an unconditional stimulus produces depolarization. He found also that through paradendritic stimulation there is a concurrent increase in the neural excitability of other cortical areas. The conditional stimulus does not produce a discharge (depolarization), but raises the excitability of the neurons by paradendritic stimulation. If these paradendritic impulses from the conditional stimulus arrive in time at a neuron when there is still an aftereffect from the unconditional stimulus, the excitability of this neuron will then be further facilitated. After repeated trials the prolonged excitation of the neuron, produced by subliminal bombardment of the paradendritic impulses, makes possible an eventual discharge with or without the combined presentation of the unconditional stimulus. Any stimulus, therefore, that impairs the function of the dendrites, or blocks the paradendritic transmissions, interferes with conditional reflex formation. According to Chang, the importance of the thalamoreticular system in the formation of the conditional reflex lies in the fact that these structures are sources of subliminal excitation of cortical neurons. He restates, however, that it is not the reticular formation, but the cortex, which performs the final integrating function in conditioning.

A complementary view to the role of the brain stem reticular formation was presented by Delgado, Grastyan, and others. Matsumoto expressed the view that besides the cortex and the ascending activating system of the brain stem the amygdaloid-hippocampal structures play a part in conditional reflex formation. Lissak postulated that these latter structures perform the inhibitory function in a controlling system of which the brain stem is the activating one.

In contrast to these views on the site of conditional reflex formation, analyzing the role of specific structures, less localized conceptions have also developed. Konorski assumed that in general the formation and multiplication of synaptic connections within the brain are at the basis of the new conditional reflex; Fessard assumed that on the polyneuronal level there is a long-lasting circulation of impulses together with redistribution of excitatory and inhibitory actions to form a new pattern. Between the extremes of the focal or too general views on the site of conditional reflex formation are the approaches based on Ukhtomski's concept of the "dominant focus," which he characterized as a relatively heightened excitability of a group of nerve cells leading to a summation of the excitations arriving from a variety of sources and a retention of this excitation once it has been established, thus leading to a capacity to continue a stable discharge when the original excitations have disappeared. The concept of dominant focus was employed in the views of John, Pribram, and others on conditional reflex formation. They quote the experiment in which conditioned avoidance response was established by pairing a metronome beat (conditional stimulus) with a shock (unconditional stimulus) to the *left rear paw* of a dog. They then placed a small piece of filter paper soaked in strychnine on the part of the motor cortex that primarily controls action of the *right forepaw*. Following strychninization, presentation of the conditional stimulus elicited vigorous flexion of the *right fore* rather than the *left rear* paw. Thus the chemically induced excitable focus dominates, and the conditional stimulus which had previously been processed on the basis of experience, in the new situation initiates a response consistent with the chemical manipulation. Jasper's findings with a monkey that was conditioned to withdraw its right arm to avoid shock, but that would withdraw the left if the signal was switched to that, supports the hypothesis that a dominant focus has an important role and is the site of conditional reflex formation.

ELECTROENCEPHALOGRAPHIC CORRELATES OF
CONDITIONAL RESPONSES

After Berger's observation that cerebral electrical potentials could be recorded through the intact skull (1929), Adrian and Matthews discovered that these electrical potentials (Berger rhythms—alpha waves) arose predominantly from the occipital lobes and were abolished when the eyes were open or if the subject concentrated on a problem (1934). Rheinberg and Jasper (1937) observed that arousal or attention results in a low-amplitude fast activity on the electroencephalogram, and Davis (1939) and Popov (1950, 1953) found that sound may also cause alpha blocking that, in contrast to light or concentration, is transient and gradually diminishes with repetition. Temporary disappearance of alpha activity also occurs whenever any stimulus is presented. By repetition of the stimulus, Sokolov (1959) distinguished between the primary startle (orienting) response, which causes generalized desynchronization with the appearance of low-amplitude fast activity diffusely over the cranium, and the secondary orienting ("what is it?") reflex, which causes a localized desynchronization in the area corresponding to the sensory modality of the stimulus. Further repetition results in disappearance of any desynchronization (Jus and Jus 1960, Roger 1960).

The first electroencephalographic evidence of a *conditioned* cerebral response is the appearance of diffuse desynchronization of the electroencephalogram in response to the conditional stimulus before the onset of the unconditional stimulus. Repetition of associated stimuli (conditional and unconditional stimuli) leads to narrowing the zone of desynchronization until it becomes limited to the region of the brain subserved by the unconditional reflex (Durup and Fessard 1935, Loomis *et al.* 1936, Travis and Egan 1938, Morrell and Jasper 1956, etc.). Although the elaboration of a cerebral conditional reflex is usually associated with a reduction of cerebral synchrony and the appearance of low-voltage fast activity over the region of the unconditional analyzer, cerebral desynchronization bears no constant relation to the behavioral conditional reflex. Repeated, non-reinforced administration of the conditional stimulus leads to extinction of the conditional reflex, which manifests in an increased cerebral synchrony during the administration of the conditional stimulus (Roitbak). Similar patterns occur with delay and differentiation (Gastaut 1956, 1957, 1958). While there is a local enhancement, increased synchrony (reappearance of alpha activity or the appearance of slow waves) in the region previously blocked by the conditional stimulus in the case of internal inhibition, external inhibition produces a generalized desynchronization or blocking of the alpha rhythm. This may correlate with Kogan's findings that desynchronization may accompany excitation or may accompany inhibition and that it is a sign of neurons at work, independently, whether this work is "excitatory" or "inhibitory."

From this review of physiological mechanisms it can be seen that two of the main known functional systems of the central nervous system, the afferent sensory and the ascending reticular system, which are strongly interconnected, are interacting during the conditioning procedure. Their connection to the third, motivational-limbic system in conditioning is achieved through the ventral part of the thalamus. The application of conditioning test procedures, therefore, promises to be rewarding in obtaining accurate information of the complex functional activity of the central nervous system, which forms the background (or physical substrata) to the different behavioral-psychological manifestations.

It can also be seen from this review that a conditional reflex is established if, and only if, the relationship between certain events is more consistent and coherent than would be expected by chance (Walter), and more recent findings have suggested that conditioned behavior is more readily established in individuals with an electroencephalogram with a large amplitude monorhythmic alpha and a higher alpha index than in those with polyrhythmic traces or low amplitude and greater spatial variation (Storm Van Leeuwen).

All the findings presented here are extensively discussed in the collected material of the Marseille (1957) and Moscow (1960) symposia and in Wells' (1961) presentation at the research conference "Electroencephalographic Correlates of Behavior" held at the Yale University School of Medicine.

PART TWO

Pavlovian Psychiatry

5

PAVLOVIAN GENERAL

PSYCHOPATHOLOGY

THE HISTORY OF scientific attempts to correlate psychopathology with pathological brain functions began in the mid-nineteenth century. From that period a long line of investigators, belonging to different schools, searched in different directions but always entertained that basic thought.

The first application of the reflex theory to psychiatry appeared at the end of the last century. Wernicke was among the prominent representatives of these earlier attempts. After his original description of sensory aphasia, he concentrated on the representation of psychological functions of the brain. The reflex arc was Wernicke's functional working unit, and he saw the cerebral cortex as the organ of "associations." In his "reflex pathology" he dealt with the three functional aspects of the reflex arc: sensory input, interneuronal associations, and motor output. He maintained that any of the three could be separately disturbed and applied this principle to psychological disturbances. He and his pupils, among them Kleist, Bonnhoeffer, and Liepmann, then tried to arrange the whole spectrum of psychiatric experience within this framework.

A similar attempt to apply the reflex theory to psychiatry was made by Lechner, who tried to explain mental phenomena on the basis of reflex action.

Pavlov's approach differed basically from that of his predecessors in the clinical field. Utilizing his own method and inferring the functions of the central nervous system from behavioral observations, he used analogies between the symptoms

51

described in patients and the different conditions observed in animals during the conditioning procedure. However, after Bekhterev's early experiments and in spite of the attempts of a large number of investigators, the application of the conditioning method in psychiatry remained for many years only a promising challenge. This impasse may be attributed to the fact that not until quite recently did neurophysiological research offer the prospect of correlating Pavlov's behavioral phenomena with processes in the central nervous system.

In Pavlov's view only a thorough, neurophysiologically based psychiatry could be called a clinical science. This view he aptly expressed in his "Letter to the Youth": "Learn the ABC's of Science before attempting to ascend its heights. Never reach for the next step without having mastered the preceding one."

Today there are many schools of psychiatry, each trying to explain from different viewpoints psychological manifestations and phenomena. The basic viewpoint of the majority is causal and deterministic. They are unanimous in dealing with the organism as a functional entity but differ in their emphasis on those properties which are biologically inherited and those which are environmentally acquired. Some stress the prominence of the affective, emotional processes. Others consider the instinctual background to be the most important.

The Pavlovian school stresses the prevailing importance to learning of experience and emphasizes the prevailing importance of the signalization process and of the crucial role played by verbal signals in thinking and communication.

In this framework, pathological symptoms are basically conditional reflex pattern alterations. Syndromes are collections of these, and psychiatric illnesses are the clinical manifestations, as they interfere with personality functioning and life adaptation.

In the definition of the normal person as one who fulfills certain demands of society and conforms to the patterns that rule interpersonal relationships, normality is used as a social term, and consequently the definition of abnormality reflects social constellations. Psychiatry, being a branch of the medical sciences that is closely allied to the social sciences, employs the term "normality" comprehensively to include the social and the physiological. Similarly, the term "pathological" refers to the unbalanced functioning of the organism in a comprehensive sense. Diseases are clinical manifestations, in which well-described psychopathology is manifest. Pavlovian psychopathology was derived from Pavlovian physiology of the highest nervous functions (psychology) and deals with the unbalance of this particular aspect of human functioning.

Sherrington considered the reflex circuit as the basic activity of the nervous system; Pavlov extended this concept to all human behavior. According to him, all reflex activity has one of two forms: unconditional or conditional. The efferent part of the reflex can be seen in the activity of a single muscle, in the well-defined activity of a group of muscles (segmental reflex), in polysegmental activity, and in locomotor acts. This reflex activity (simple reflexes, autonomic activity, unconditional movements) may reach higher levels of integration in more complex unconditional reflexes (emotional, instinctual stereotypes). The highest level or organization is reached in consciously directed voluntary co-ordinations.

Initiation of a reflex is always due to a stimulus, either external or internal, physical, chemical, verbal, or psychological. As with the reflexes, stimuli also may belong to one of two groups: unconditional or conditional. Unconditional reflexes by heredity utilize a specific response pattern (from single muscle activity to the instinctual stereotypes). In the development of the organism other agents, inessential and previously ineffective, become associated with the stereotyped unconditional (stimulus-response) connections. The process of functional adaptation is made possible by the widening number and variations of possible stimulations that elicit response and is promoted by the coupling, or associating, capacity of the nervous system, which links the new environmental or internal stimuli with the effector components of the unconditional reflexes. The resulting newly developed conditional reflexes *promote* an extremely varied orientation and adaptation to the environment, through the consciously directed voluntary co-ordinations and automatisms, which constitutes, according to Pavlov, the unified first signal system of the organism.

In humans another system of signaling is added, by means of which signals of the first system may be signaled. In this signaling, the conditional stimulus of a well-established conditional reflex serves as the unconditional stimulus of a consecutive conditional reflex. This second conditional stimulus (secondary in order to the first conditional stimulus) is speech, in which verbal signals are utilized. A verbal signal (word symbol), by continuous association with its adequate primary signal complex, in time becomes the conditional stimulus of the primary signal complex. By means of this primary signal complex the word symbol achieves a connection with the unconditional effector apparatus. Since, in these constellations, secondary conditional stimuli signal primary conditional stimuli, the whole of these complexes was called by Pavlov the second signal system. These verbal signals may elicit responses similar to those of any other physical or chemical, unconditional or conditional stimuli. Through these signals both the outer and the inner world are extensively perceived. While the human being regularly receives varied unconditional and conditional (primary and secondary) stimuli, it frequently occurs that the secondary conditional stimuli begin to prevail.

Pavlov viewed the process of functional adaptation typologically. Depending on whether the primary or secondary conditional stimulus elicits greater response, or, in other words, depending on whether the first or second signal systems prevail, Pavlov saw within the normal range three groups: artists, with a predominating first signal system; thinkers, with a prevailing second signal system; and a middle group with equal proportions of both.

Within the foregoing frame of reference Pavlov's general psychopathology deals with all three psychological structural organizations: the cognitive, the relational, and the adaptive. These three structures are, in fact, aspects of the three sections of the reflex arc. From the afferent part comes the perceptual and cognitive structure; from the central part, the relational; and from the efferent part, the adaptive.

The primary phenomenon of the cognitive structure is the diffuse sensation produced by an impulse. The impulse is conducted by the sensory nerves from the external and internal world to the central nervous system, where the created sensations are synthesized into perception. While sensations are the most elementary psychophysiological processes, perceptions arise when the new sensations ecphorize traces of similar former sensations. When we see an object, it vividly and distinctly appears in our consciousness with all its concrete features. We perceive it in the environment, where it—without doubt—really exists. We cannot deliberately change the content of this perception because it is determined by the characteristics of the object that, through our sense organs, acts on the analyzer of the brain. Such stimulation sensation of the analyzers gives rise to perceptions. Concepts, on the other hand, are the "recollected mental images of perceptions." Thus perception is based on direct environmental stimulation of the cerebral analyzers, while a concept is based on weak traces of stimulation retained at the same locus. According to Pavlov, hallucinations arise if these weak traces of former stimulations grow abnormally strong in some part of the brain, causing excitation. They attain various degrees of intensity up to the force of real perceptions. These perceptions without corresponding stimuli from outside or inside are called hallucinations.

Before Pavlov, Kandinsky, in his principal work on pseudo-hallucinations, described hallucinations as imaginary perceptions. They closely resembled dreams. Consequently, he defined dreams as hallucinations in sleep and hallucinations as dreams occurring while awake. He found that most of the characteristics of dreams are also typical of hallucinations; in both we deal with imaginary perceptions, that is, perceptions of what does not really exist. In Kandinsky's view hallucinations arise in connection with a local excitation in the cerebral cortex (in the cerebral center of some sense organ) with a simultaneous general exhaustion of the other parts of the cortex. Popov elaborated on Kandinsky's concept, utilizing Pavlov's frame of reference. His experiments showed that the inhibitory phenomena that lead to hypnotic phases (equalized and paradoxical) have a promoting role in the appearance of hallucinations. This finding was supported by the fact that some drugs that evoke and strengthen inhibition may foster the appearance of hallucinations.

In the paradoxical phase of sleep (inhibition) there is a strong reaction to a weak stimulation. In hallucination the relatively weak traces of former sensations (perceptions) become dominant and induce a greater effect than the "concrete" stimuli of the environment.

The highest level of the cognitive psychological organization is thinking. The mental derangements, on this level, for which Pavlov put forward physiological explanations, were obsessions and delusions.

Obsessions are ideas that continually obtrude in the foreground, against the individual's will. They obtrude with or without a known external or internal cause. Pavlov characterized obsessions and compulsions as excessively stable ideas, manifested in thinking and in actions, respectively. In his view their pathophysiological basis lies in an increased inertness of excitation in isolated, pathodynamic structures of the cerebral hemispheres.

In describing the role of the conditional reflexes in the fine adjustment of the organism to the constantly changing environment, Rokhlin pointed out the signaling nature of the conditional stimuli, the significance of the temporary bounds established by them, and the importance of their "signal significance." If the stimulus loses its "signal significance" and changes from a true to a false signal, the response reaction formerly elaborated to it may become superfluous or harmful. In such cases inhibition of these conditional reflexes comes to the fore. Under normal circumstances the permanently interacting excitatory and inhibitory processes determine behavior and help in forming an equilibrium with the environment, that is, they adjust the activity of the organism to the changing life conditions. In obsession this equilibrium is impaired, since the increased inertness of the excitatory process impedes the inhibition of the reflexes, which have lost their signal significance. Since at the basis of this process there is an increased inertness of excitation with a concomitant weak inhibition—a result of paradoxical induction—in the surrounding areas, the latter cannot suppress the cerebral activity of the other physiologically functioning parts of the brain, to which the conceptions opposed to the obsession are connected. Hence the insight of the obsessive patient.

Delusions are classically defined as incorrect ideas, created not by an accidental insufficiency of logic but out of an inner need, which Kraepelin called the "delusional need." Thus delusions are expressed in erroneous judgments arising on a morbid basis and appearing perfectly reasonable to the patient.

The Pavlovian concepts on the origin of delusions is best explained by Rokhlin through a concrete example. The patient is suffering from persecutory delusions and insists that his sister and mother want to kill him. He is certain of this idea, though his relatives display all possible concern for him and are hurt by his unjust accusations. In Pavlovian terms this patient's judgment is determined "by his higher nervous activity which is altered by the illness and is in the ultraparadoxical phase" (of sleep inhibition). Therefore the real, strong stimuli—the facts of life, that is, his relatives' concern for him—fail to be correspondingly reflected in his brain; the cerebral activity that normally would call for the correspondingly correct thoughts is not excited. Nor are the weaker stimulations in the brain—underlying the wrong idea—inhibited. On the contrary, these latter stimuli acquire greater force and contribute to the stability of the delusion.

Pavlov conceived delusions as the result of two coinciding psychological phenomena: the ultraparadoxical hypnotic phase and the increased inertness of excitation. In the concrete example quoted, this ultraparadoxical hypnotic phase is seen in the fact that the usually inhibitory influences—the weaker stimulations underlying the ideas opposite to reality—produce the reverse effect, that is, evoke excitation. The force and stability of this delusion thus is based on the increased inertness of excitation in an isolated pathodynamic structure of the brain connected with the delusion. This produces sufficiently strong inhibition of the cerebral activity with the realistic antagonistic ideas, around the strong but inert focus of excitation. The pathodynamic structure with the increased inertness of excitation is isolated in the brain, which explains how the patient retains sober judgment in other problems of life.

In both obsession and delusion there is an increased inertness of excitation at isolated pathodynamic cerebral structures. But, while Pavlov believed that in obsession the force of this increased inertness of excitation is less pronounced and therefore cannot fully inhibit the cerebral activity with which the conceptions opposed to the obsession are connected (and therefore a critical attitude and some insight are retained), in delusion the force of this increased inertness of excitation is particularly great, and therefore a strong inhibition arises around the pathodynamic structures in the brain that retards the activity of the cerebrum where the appropriate ideas (insight) opposed to the delusion are connected.

Pavlov also discussed the dynamics of these pathologic processes (hallucinations, obsessions, delusions). He believed that irregular development or a disease of an organ may cause strong excitation in the brain. Such a condition would precipitate a pathologically increased inertness of the excitatory process, which would manifest itself in an irresistible concept (on a lower level an irresistible perception) continuing even after its cause has been withdrawn. Strong, overwhelming life experiences may have the same result. Most of the pathological inertness of excitation seen is due to this cause, since "human life is an incessant struggle between aspirations, wishes and tastes, and the general, natural and social conditions." Depending upon the level of pathologically increased inertness of excitation, the pathological process or psychopathological functioning may be found in areas that receive immediate stimulation from external and internal agents (first signal system), or, alternatively, it may be found in different areas of the verbal system (second signal system). In both cases the pathological inertness of excitation produces pathological symptoms, perceptual alterations (hallucinations and pseudohallucinations), and alterations of thinking (obsessions and delusions), respectively.

The concepts of psychopathology of the relational—emotional—structural organization have also been adapted to this physiological framework. It is based on the observation of animals after the removal of their cerebral hemispheres and of humans under the influence of narcotics. The waking, active cortex produces negative inductions in the subcortex. It is an inhibitory state of the cortex that produces a positive induction in the subcortical centers, intensifying its general activity. This weakness of the cortex is manifested in a special state called "emotional lability" and in actions affected directly by the subcortical centers. Such actions are produced under the influence of a tendency without preliminary control and were called "affective" or "emotional" by Pavlov.

The psychopathology of mood, which also belongs to the relational—affective—structure, is based on observations from the period during which Pavlov was working with dynamic stereotypes. According to Pavlov, depressed feelings are experienced at times of a change in the "general mode of living." This depression has its physiological basis in the extinction of the old dynamic stereotype, along with difficulty in establishing a new one. The resulting state of change shows first an increased anxiety and tension, which may then decompensate into a depressed mood or neurotic illness.

Finally, there is the adaptive structural organization, which represents all our activity psychophysiologically (manifest behavior). The adaptive organization—or apparatus—is determined by the effect of the conditional reflexes and unconditional reflexes. It is influenced by central volitional, or subcortical, activity or by the hypnotic states.

Pavlovian psychopathology, therefore, presents the human psyche as an entity that can, however, be artificially divided into cognitive, relational, and adaptive structures (Nyirö).

Superimposed and correlating the functions of these structures is consciousness, of which attention and memory are integral parts. Herbart defined consciousness as the sum of all

real or simultaneously present ideas, while Wundt saw it as
the association of the psychological structures. Bleuler considered consciousness to be indefinable in itself but to be that
quality which most clearly differentiates us from the autom-
aton. Others viewed it as a reflexion of the material and
being. Nyirö elaborated Jasper's concepts, describing consciousness as the highest synthetical function of the nervous
system, which makes it possible to recognize the external and
the internal world and its influences and occurrences.

Consciousness, according to Pavlov, is the nervous activity
of a certain part of the cerebral hemispheres, which possesses
at a given moment optimal excitability with a maximal excitatory state, the excitability and the excitatory state of the peripheral parts of the cerebral hemispheres being diminished at
the same time. The center of the optimal excitability is the
conscious, creative part of the hemispheres. At this point new
conditional reflexes are easily formed and differentiation is
successfully developed. In the peripheral, unconscious part,
because of decreased excitability, even previously elaborated
reflexes function in a lower, stereotyped fashion. The area of
optimal excitability perpetually migrates.

Attention, according to Bleuler, is a manifestation of affectivity, in which certain sensory perceptions and ideas that have
aroused our interest are facilitated, while all others are inhibited. Recent definitions describe attention as that constellation of the consciousness in which sensorial perceptions are
foremost.

Attention is a complex psychic function. Its elemental functions are concentration, tenacity, and vigilance. Concentration
is the ability to exclude all associations irrelevant to a certain
theme. In a positive sense it can be measured by the quantity
of relevant associations to a certain theme within a certain
time. Tenacity is the ability to keep one's attention focused on
a certain subject continuously, and vigilance is the capacity to
direct one's attention to a new subject. In Pavlovian terms
concentration is manifested in the number of conditional connections simultaneously present, tenacity in the persistence of
these conditional connections, and vigilance in their mobility.

Memories are based on acquired conditional connections retained in the brain.

Other factors that influence the prevailing forms of the symptoms of an illness are related to the dynamic relationship between the patient's constitutional type, or temperament (personality), and the strength and type of the acting stimuli from the external or internal world.

Depending on the strength of the nervous system, beyond a certain maximal intensity of stimulation, there may be variations in responses, leading to equivalent, paradoxical, or ultra-paradoxical rather than proportional responses. In such a manner an ultramaximal stimulus may result in various degrees of inhibition (hypnotic state). Furthermore, Pavlov stressed that, whereas in the inhibitory type a strong stimulus considerably weakens the excitatory process (producing an inhibited state), in the excitable type such stimuli weaken the inhibitory process and result in excitation.

Strong functional interrelation exists between all the psychic faculties described (cognitive, relational, adaptive; reflected in consciousness and manifested in personality) and also between the other somatic and autonomic (physical) faculties. Dissociation among them and regression of any of them from a higher to a lower level is the principal territory with which clinical psychiatry concerns itself.

6

PAVLOVIAN CLINICAL PSYCHOPATHOLOGY

THE CONCEPTS of the Pavlovian brain model and of general psychopathology were applied clinically, primarily in the study of the neuroses but also in the study of the psychoses. They led to therapeutic implications.

NEUROSES

Following the early presentation by Pavlov and Shenger-Krestovnikova of a condition resembling human neurosis that could be experimentally induced in animals, the interest in experimental neurosis increased greatly. The Pavlovian school (Petrova, Rickman, and Gantt, among others) contributed greatly to the concept from the physiological viewpoint. Gantt brought early recognition of the concept beyond the confines of Europe when he introduced it to North America. In psychiatric circles, Masserman, among others, saw the importance of the existence of a method that might be able to produce a condition resembling human neurosis, recognizing the importance of the fact that under experimental conditions the pathomechanisms and manifestations of neurosis could be studied. In his biologically oriented, dynamic approach he put forward the Pavlovian concept in a broader sense and felt that, by inducing two conflicting motivations, the resulting behavior could justifiably be called neurotic.

Pavlov's concepts of the experimental neuroses developed in three stages (Wells). In the first stage of the work it was found that it was possible to induce "nervous breakdown" in the two extreme types of dogs, that is, the weak inhibitory and the strong excitatory, by means of conflicting or of excessively strong (powerful) stimuli. Typical of the experiments in the first stage were those of Petrova and Rickman.

Petrova used dogs belonging to the two extreme types and elaborated in each dog six conditional reflexes in which the response was delayed for three minutes. Thereafter, she confronted the animals with a strong electric stimulus, which ordinarily would evoke an unconditional defensive reaction. Instead of the withdrawal reaction, the dogs were to develop a conditioned food response, that is, licking the feeding dish. Both dogs accomplished this, but, with the increasing strength of the electric shock in the dog with the weak inhibitory type of nervous system, all previously elaborated positive conditional reflexes disappeared and the animal became extremely sleepy, while in the other dog, of the strong excitable type, all previously elaborated inhibitory reactions were lost and his behavior was highly excited. Several months of rest brought about a complete cure of the inhibitory neurosis, while the excitatory neurosis was eliminated only by giving 2 per cent potassium bromide rectally.

Rickman in his experiment used dogs belonging to the weak inhibitory type. He applied simultaneously the following stimuli: a loud cracking sound, sudden presentation of a grotesque mask and a fur coat turned inside out, an explosion of gunpowder near the stand, and a special swinging platform mounted on the stand on which the dog was placed. The dog rushed forward immediately and then became completely rigid. To account for this behavior, it was assumed that there was a general inhibition (transmarginal or protective inhibition), which was accompanied by the disappearance of all the conditional and unconditional food reflexes and which lasted, with fluctuations, for sixteen days. This inhibitory neurosis, which was produced by too strong (overpowering) stimuli, recurred six months later in one of the dogs as a result of flood and a great hurricane.

On the basis of these experiments it was assumed that

there are two stressful situations that lead to neurosis in the animal, that only the extreme, unbalanced type of animal is susceptible to neurosis, and, furthermore, that the character of the neurosis depends mainly on the type of the animal's nervous system.

In the second stage, work was directed to expose the animal to various stressful situations. Among them were the administration of extremely strong stimuli, elaboration of extremely delicate differentiations, the development of a conditional reflex to every fourth stimulus, the quick transition of a negative stimulus into a positive and a positive into a negative one, and a change in the previously established order of conditional stimuli (dynamic stereotype). On the basis of these experiments Pavlov concluded that, besides overstrain of the excitatory process and/or the inhibitory process, an overstrain of the mobility of the nervous processes may also lead to pathological stages. During this period it became obvious that the dependence of the possibility of breakdown and of the character of the breakdown on the type of higher nervous activity could no longer be held to be absolute but, on the contrary, was considered to be highly relative. It was also in this period that the idea that there are really two forms of neuroses, the excitatory and the inhibitory, was no longer tenable. First, it was found that the excitatory neuroses are often accompanied by one or another of the hypnotic phases (mixed neurosis). Then it was discovered that inhibitory neuroses are also frequently accompanied by motor excitement. Finally, it was revealed that sometimes an abrupt transition from an excitatory neurosis to an inhibitory neurosis takes place. Thus in the second stage of the work considerable broadening and differentiation of the theory took place.

Finally, in the third stage, work was concentrated on changes resulting from overstrain of mobility. It was during this period that the "isolated pathological points" or "isolated pathodynamic structures" were described as a consequence mainly of an abrupt change in the dynamic stereotype. This led to the discovery of two additional mechanisms of functional disturbances: pathological inertness and pathological lability, at opposite poles from each other. In the case of pathological inertness conditional reflexes cannot be changed or extinguished, while in pathological lability certain conditional reflexes cannot be fixed, are highly unstable, and are constantly changing. Pathological inertness leads to mechanical repetition of responses, while pathological lability leads to chaotic behavior. It was also in this period that it was revealed that isolated pathodynamic structures have a tendency to spread to other dynamic structures of the brain.

Thus the Pavlovian concept of experimental neuroses was based on observations in animal experiments. It was based on the findings that certain deviations from the normal may develop without the presence of an extraneous pathological agent.

In the human neuroses Pavlov saw also a psychological reaction to exogenous factors. His definition agrees with the teachings of classical German psychiatry, which recognized and described sharp distinctions between faulty development, manifested in mental deficiency and psychopathy; endogenous psychoses of unknown etiology, such as manic-depressive psychoses and schizophrenia; and reaction types to an exogenous traumatic factor, organic or psychological, such as dementia paralytica and the neuroses. In viewing the etiology of neuroses Pavlov considered the same exogenous factors at work as in the etiology of the experimental neuroses of the animal. On the other hand, Pavlov classified humans on the basis of their biologically conditioned temperament (choleric, sanguine, phlegmatic, and melancholic) and classified them also on an environmentally conditioned basis (as artists and thinkers). In neurasthenia the alteration induced by the exogenous factor is general, and only the order of its development differs, depending on the biologically conditioned temperamental type.

In other neurotic conditions the reaction is dependent on the environmentally conditioned basis. For example, in the case of artists (with a dominance of first signal system experiences), the neurotic reaction is seen in hysteria. In the case of thinkers, with a predominance of second signal system experiences, it is seen in psychasthenia. In all forms of neuroses

there is a stress-organism interaction, to which the organism
reacts defensively. The starting point of the reaction is dependent on the specific biological and environmental constellation,
leading under continuous stress to a hypnotic state. In this
manner, according to Pavlov, the neuroses not only are quantitatively different from the psychoses but also show a definite
qualitative difference. Thus psychoses are, by his system,
beyond the scope of being induced by a quantitatively overwhelming environmental stimulation and represent situations
in which a definite, third, pathological factor is added.

Pavlov's concept of the importance of types in human
neuroses correlated with the findings of a number of different
dynamically oriented psychiatric schools. Szondi, for instance,
had found in a type of neurosis (neurasthenia) illnesses of
different kinds, depending on the constitutional type.

Pavlov's concepts attracted notice, and even Schilder (then
already psychoanalytically oriented) remarked, in an article
on the somatic basis of the neurosis, that all the symptoms of
human neurosis could be found in Pavlov's experimentally produced neurosis of dogs. Schilder, however, denied that it would
ever be possible to understand and explain human neurosis
fully on the basis of Pavlov's findings. As a reaction to Pavlov's
findings, he expressed his belief that all the symptoms of the
experimentally induced neurosis of the dog could be understood and explained by the psychological mechanisms of the
analytical school.

In his reply to Schilder, Pavlov re-emphasized his concept.
He stressed that the meaning of any interpretation in science
is based on increasingly refined observations, by means of
which elements of the complex can be integrated. Consequently, one should not try to understand the analogous manifestations of the animal neurosis in terms of the human psyche,
but, rather, the interpretation of the human neurosis should be
helped by an understanding of the mechanisms brought to
light in the manifestations of the experimentally induced
animal neurosis.

Pavlov also clarified some further points in his reply. He
emphasized the importance of determining, and, even more,

of qualifying, the way in which behavior of neurotics differs from that of normals. Granting neurosis to be a reaction to exogenous factors, he also stressed the necessity of determining, from the patient's history, those elements to which the neurosis could be etiologically connected and also those elements which might contribute to the actual pathological symptoms, for example, the temperamental type. Furthermore, Pavlov stressed the importance, as a first step, of studying the actual changes that take place in the nervous system in correlation with these neurotic symptoms rather than theorizing on unknown psychodynamic mechanisms.

In his appraisal of Freud's theory Pavlov made similar remarks:

> When I think of Freud and of us physiologists I have in mind two parties of miners who began to drive a tunnel at the foot of a big mountain in order to bring to light—the understanding of the human mind. But Freud started digging downward and has dug himself into the labyrinth of the unconscious, whereas we shall some time come out into the open, into the air and light, and shall finish building the tunnel. We are certain to finish it because we are on the right track. By studying the relationship between the cortex and the subcortex we are already able to show the ways nervous processes, both conscious and subconscious develop; we have established phenomena of cortical induction, have learned to reproduce the neuroses and have joined the clinic to physiology, while Freud is only trying to guess the inner states of man.

Pavlov then applied his method to the investigation of human neuroses and analyzed and interpreted in detail the three prevailing forms of neurosis of his time, neurasthenia, hysteria, and psychasthenia, by correlating his observations and knowledge in the psychiatric field with his findings in animal experiments. The forms of neurosis that are more common nowadays, for example, obsessive-compulsive neurosis, neurotic depression, etc., he treated less extensively.

Neurasthenia

The condition that had been described as "nervosisme" was introduced in America under the name of "neurasthenia" by Beard (1869), who thought that a weak mental Anlage, which is an inherited disposition or response pattern of the individual to exogenous stress, is the necessary predisposing factor in this illness (1880). He received further support in this regard from Janet (1908).

Another view of the condition was presented by Arndt (1892). According to him, neurasthenia represents to a certain degree the starting point of all the more severe nervous disorders. Similarly, Stertz (1928) considered neurasthenia the mildest form of cerebral illness and pointed out that organic diseases frequently present neurasthenic symptoms in their early stages. This view was closely related to that of Bonnhoeffer, who saw in neurasthenia a non-specific reaction to different traumatizing stimulations (i.e., toxic, etc.), which produced, clinically, emotional hyperesthesia, irritability, weakness, and nervousness.

The concept was further elaborated by Freud, who in his early writings considered neurasthenia as a form of the actual neuroses (1900). He wrote: "Psychoneuroses appear under two kinds of conditions, either independently or in the wake of the actual neuroses: neurasthenia or anxiety neurosis." Later on, Ferenczi referred to the actual neuroses as physioneuroses, in contrast to the psychoneuroses (1908).

This was the state of affairs when Pavlov presented his views on neurasthenia, which he developed in three stages. In the first stage he induced neurosis experimentally in dogs of the "excitable" type. The animals lost all their inhibitory reflexes, while retaining their positive conditional reflexes. This condition reminded Pavlov of human neurasthenia, which he considered at this point a specific illness of the "excitable" animal.

In the second stage Pavlov induced neurosis experimentally both in "excitable" strong and "inhibited" weak animals. The neurosis was manifested in the disappearance of the inhibitory reflexes and of the positive conditional reflexes, respectively.

The former group of animals responded favorably, the latter group unfavorably, to the treatment with bromides. Since, to Pavlov, both these conditions resembled human neurasthenia, he revised his former views and named the neurasthenia of the excitable type "hypersthenia" and of the inhibited type "hyposthenia." At this point he considered hypersthenia and hyposthenia as distinct disease entities.

In the third stage of experimentation Pavlov found that animals that first presented hypersthenic manifestations later, under continued stress, "changed" and presented a hyposthenic picture. On the basis of these findings he concluded that neurasthenia is not restricted to a specific temperamental type, that only the manifestations of the initial phase are constitutionally determined, and that hyper- and hyposthenia are not two independent diseases but two consecutive phases of the same disease.

The Pavlovian concepts of neurasthenia were applied to human psychopathology by Ivanov-Smolensky. He surmised on the basis of clinical observations and experiments that neurasthenia develops in three stages. In the first stage the most recent and vulnerable processes of internal inhibition are impaired, in the second stage the excitatory process also becomes involved, and in the third stage protective inhibition sets in.

On the basis of this pathological process, the hypersthenic manifestations, initial irritability (emotional hyperesthesia, overreaction, sensitive reaction, nervousness), can be correlated with the impairment of internal inhibitory reflexes, that is, impairment of reflex delay, and so on.

The weakness and, in general, the hyposthenic manifestations, the constant feeling of exhaustion, and the generalized psychological and physical asthenia can all be correlated with the condition produced when conditioning ability is reduced and when conditional reflexes can be formed only with difficulty.

Finally, the further stress-induced, quantitative, stimulus-response alteration is due to the hypnotic state. The protective inhibition thus produced is the result of an extreme stress.

Regarding the etiology of neurasthenia in humans, Pavlov

thought that it is brought about by physical and psychical exhaustion, by highly charged emotional situations or conflicts. He maintained that many prominent people had been neurasthenic and emphasized that people suffering from neurasthenia may still be able to carry on a large amount of activity and accomplish much in life.

Hysteria

The Greek term "hysteria" means wandering of the uterus. Pericles claimed its relation to sexual disturbance, which view was supported by Hippocrates. For many centuries hysteria was believed to be a specific illness of the female.

However, despite the controversy in etiology (Scholastic: heart; Gallenic: brain), hysterical states are seen as those in which some motivation in the background of the physical or psychological symptoms can be found. Hysteria can mimic almost any disease and manifests itself in innumerable forms.

The modern concepts of hysteria began with Charcot, who described the typical clinical picture, which could also be induced by hypnosis. Furthermore, Charcot thought of hypnosis itself as a solely hysterical phenomenon, meaning that only hysterics could be hypnotized. Both views were disproved (Liebault, Bernheim, Babinsky, etc.). Pavlov's concepts of hysteria were based on Charcot's but also on Janet's views, who saw in hysteria a physical disorder, resulting from weakness and especially from "exhaustion" of the brain.

A third source for Pavlov's theory were Jackson's hierarchical concepts: the three organizational levels in which the higher level exerts control over the lower. Pavlov believed that the cerebral cortex, being at the highest organizational level, constantly controls the lower emotional, instinctual, and other activities, which have their center in the subcortical areas. This physiological control, exerted by the cerebral cortex, diminishes in the case of a "weak mental Anlage." It diminishes even more when this weakness is potentiated by one of the factors that exhausts the brain. The diminished control results in chaotic functioning (seen in emotional, instinctual, stereotypic functioning) at the released lower level. The chaotic activity is even further potentiated by positive induction, one of the basic patterns of functioning of the central nervous system. Continuous cortical analytical and synthetic functioning (well-balanced excitatory and inhibitory processes) in the waking, active state produces negative induction in the subcortex as the result of excitation that is due to continuously received external and internal stimuli. Consequently, subcortical activity is restrained by paradoxically induced inhibition. In hysteria the weakened and exhausted nervous system cannot cope proportionately any longer with the external or internal stimulations. Under increasing stress the proportionate stimulus-response relationship becomes altered, and one of the "hypnotic" states sets in. In this, the inhibitory process prevails. In hysteria this prevailing inhibitory process of the cortex, in accordance with the pattern of reciprocal induction, now produces a positive induction of the subcortical centers. As a result, hysterical manifestations appear, which under normal circumstances are kept under control by negative induction.

Furthermore, Pavlov thought of the pathology that underlies the clinical manifestations in hysteria as the morbid predominance of the first signal system over the second. Thus the artistic type is predisposed to this illness and may respond to an overstrain with the predominance of the sensory-perceptual system over the speech system, of emotional responses over rational thought. With the disappearance of the normally regulating second signal system influences, the activity of the first signal system becomes chaotic (characterized by pathological fantasies and emotional behavior). The permanent emotional excitation produces overstrain leading to protective inhibition. This passes through the various hypnotic phases of equalization, paradoxical and ultraparadoxical, with their particular clinical syndromes: suggestibility, catalepsy, twilight states, anesthesia, and paralysis (Wells).

According to Pavlov, hysteria is similar to any other neurosis. It is a reaction to an exogenous psychological or physical factor. However, while in neurasthenia—which is the illness of the excitable type—the prominent symptoms (stages of the condition) are at first manifested in the imbalance of excitatory and inhibitory phenomena and hypnotic phenomena enter only in the final stage, in hysteria, which is the illness of the inhibited type, hypnotic phenomena prevail in the clinical picture.

Pavlov's concepts of the role of protective inhibition in the symptom formation of hysterics closely resemble Freud's early concepts, that "the existence of hypnotic states forms the foundation and condition of hysteria. If such hypnotic states exist before the manifest illness they provide a foothold upon which affect establishes itself with its pathogenic recollection and its subsequent somatic manifestations."

Psychasthenia

The term "psychasthenia" was introduced as a nosological entity by Janet (1908) and referred to the neurosis that he considered the opposite of hysteria in its manifestations. The diagnosis of psychasthenia is losing favor (Hinzie and Shatsky), and in more recent times mention of it has been confined to historical interest in Western psychiatric literature (Mayer-Gross; Noyes).

Pavlov, however, elaborated upon Janet's view. He attempted to understand psychasthenia on the basis of a disturbed equilibrium between the first and second signal systems. In the "over-realism" of the psychasthenic patient, in his multiple anxieties and the intensiveness of his inhibitions, which overrule his instinctual-emotional life, Pavlov recognized the dominance of the second signal system in the disturbed equilibrium. Therefore the Pavlovian concept of psychasthenia refers to a condition in which stimuli (physical, psychological, or verbal) elicit an ideational response, the opposite to hysteria, in which the same stimuli elicit a physical response.

Psychasthenia as a form of neurosis is the result of the organism-environmental interaction to an overwhelming stimulation. According to Pavlov, the same stress that in the excitable type results in neurasthenia, in the inhibited type, in the case of dominant first signal system, leads to hysteria, while in the case of prevailing second signal system it produces psychasthenia.

Phobic Reactions

In his address to the Paris Psychological Association in 1925 Pavlov presented his view that "normal timidity, cowardice and especially pathological phobias are based on a mere predominance of the physiological process of inhibition." Ten years later at the Second International Congress in London he elaborated upon this statement by presenting Petrova's experimental findings.

Petrova's dog, which previously took its food in any situation, even at the edge of a staircase, under an experimentally induced stressful situation ceased to do so, hurriedly avoided the food, and moved away from the edge. Pavlov interpreted this as follows:

> When a normal animal, approaching the edge of a staircase stops and does not move farther, this means that it is able confidently to hold itself back, as much as is necessary to prevent it from falling down. In our case this retention is exaggerated: the reaction to depth is excessive and keeps the dog, to the detriment of its interests, much farther from the edge of the staircase than is actually necessary. Subjectively this is an obvious state of dread or fear, a phobia of depth.

Further clarification was given by Pavlov in his *Lectures on the Activity of the Cerebral Hemispheres.* Here he described a dog that normally remained awake in the experimental situation and ate the food given after the application of the conditional stimulus. By repetitive administrations of the weak conditional stimulus, a hypnotic state was induced and the dog was almost immobilized. Then a strong conditional stimulus was administered. In response, at first the dog turned to the place where the food was served and thereafter sharply turned away and did not touch the food. The dog behaved like a person who is afraid of something. As soon as the hypnotic state was eliminated, all the conditional stimuli evoked the normal effect. On the basis of these findings Pavlov felt justified in considering phobias as "natural inhibitory symptoms" of the pathologically weakened nervous system.

Transferring the findings in animal experiments to humans, and observing that phobic symptoms are prevailingly present in thinkers (subjects with a dominant second signal system), Pavlov considered phobic reactions as a specific form of psychasthenia.

Neurotic Depressions

One of the first descriptions of melancholia is to be found in the Old Testament (Saul suffered from it), while the word "melancholia" (black bile) was coined by Hippocrates. Aretaeus described the sad, listless, helpless victims of melancholia, who "complain of a thousand futilities and desire death."

Pavlov saw neurotic depression as the result of changes in the patient's customary mode of living. The customary mode of living of a person is based physiologically on well-established dynamic stereotypes. In this manner Pavlov saw the pathodynamics of neurotic depression in the destruction of this old dynamic stereotype, with the resulting difficulty in establishing a new one.

In a normal, healthy person the establishment of a new dynamic stereotype after destruction of the old one is promptly achieved. For certain neurotics, however, as part of their neurotic pattern, the period needed to establish a new dynamic stereotype becomes extended. This prolonged difficulty creates anxiety and leads to a subjective feeling of depression. At this point the stressful situation induces hypnotic mechanisms.

Psychosomatic Neuroses

Pavlov, in his book entitled *Work of the Digestive Glands,* emphasized that the activity of the main digestive glands (i.e., liver, pancreas, gastric glands) can be influenced through their nerve supply. While working with blood circulation, Pavlov became interested in the nervous regulation of the activity of the organism and developed the principle he called *nervism*, an attempt to extend the influence of the nervous system to the greatest possible number of functions of the organism. The idea was not new but had been expressed by only a few predecessors (Beard, Botkin, Feuchtersleben, Sechenov, Tsyon, etc.).

The basis of corticovisceral and viscerocortical influences is the fact that there is a neural connection between the internal organs and the cerebral cortex. This is the morphological substrate that transmits the information in both directions. Through these nerves the cerebral cortex regulates the activity of the other organs and receives information on their condition and activity. The afferent aspects (viscerocortical functioning) were already studied by Sechenov, who found that the "dark" (visceral) sensations that arrive at the brain from the internal organs play a part in the formation of man's feeling, mood, and mental activity. Korsakov added to this concept while working with hypochondriac patients whose illness he believed to be based on hyperesthesia, an increased sensitivity of the perceptors in the internal organs (Rokhlin).

Further contribution in this direction was made in Pavlov's laboratory, where it was demonstrated at first that the cerebral cortex reacts to vegetative-endocrine changes. In normal animals in the periods of heat, pregnancy, and lactation, marked functional changes were found, manifested in decreased conditioning ability, an instability of conditional reflexes, drowsiness, changes of cortical excitability, diffuse inhibition, and so on. The changes were reversible; they disappeared when the period of heat, pregnancy, or lactation was over. Similar observations were made under pathological disturbances (i.e., castration, extirpation of other glands, etc.). Immediately following castration, changes took place in all three properties (force, equilibrium, and mobility) of the basic processes. In spite of the fact that it was possible to attain full recovery of the higher nervous activity, the animals remained more susceptible to neuroses. Giliarovsky, Krasnushkin, and others transferred the work in animal laboratories to the human clinics. Astvatsaturov presented the idea that characteristic mental traits are associated with disorders of the internal organs, for example, sudden heart conditions have a concomitant sense of fear, liver damage goes with irritability.

In all the foregoing, disturbances of higher nervous activity caused by disturbances in the functioning of the internal organs have been described. In the following, influences in the opposite direction, that is, the corticovisceral, will be discussed.

Pavlov's work in the corticovisceral area of research was devoted particularly to the study of the nerves that regulate heart activity. He described the trophic cardiac nerves and indicated that they have a regulatory influence on the innervation of the heart muscles. Pavlov's idea of trophic innervation was further elaborated by Orbeli, who later named one of the functions of the sympathetic nervous system as the adaptational trophic function.

Animal experiments on corticovisceral influences were made by Bykov, Petrova, Asratyan, Usievich, and others. Petrova produced neuroses artificially in dogs. She observed that long-lasting pathological nervous activity was accompanied by various diseases of the skin, joints, kidneys, etc. Some of the animals even developed tumors. By rest, sleep, or drugs, Petrova normalized nervous activity, and a recovery of the physical condition followed. Similar observations were made by Usievich, who described biliary colic and high blood pressure accompanying the experimentally induced neurosis. This was an extension of the hypothesis of corticovisceral influences. A further step was the discovery that the condition of the cerebral cortex plays a part in the origin of diseases and also in the restoration of the normal activity disturbed by disease and injury. Speransky was among the first to claim that many diseases that had been thought local and independent of the central nervous system were caused by disturbances in the activity of various nerve centers.

Asratyan demonstrated the effect of the cerebral cortex in restoring the functions of various organs. He injured several nerves alone or together with the cerebral cortex and found that the functional recovery of the animals with an intact cortex was faster.

On the basis of these findings a new theory was elaborated. This corticovisceral theory was strengthened by the discovery that visceral functioning can definitely be conditioned. If it can be conditioned, its conditional reflex pattern may become altered even to the extent of a pathological alteration. With the assumption that, in the human, words, verbally expressed material, can become secondary conditional signals, their effect on visceral functioning can then be assumed.

The most elaborate work in this field was done by Bykov and his collaborators. He summarized their work in a book entitled *The Cerebral Cortex and Internal Organs*. The starting point of Bykov's investigation was that modern physiology had collected a vast amount of material on the organs and was now approaching the "true central problem," the physiology of the individual cell and its significance to the whole organism. According to him, to control or influence a specific organ of the human organism, one must know the conditions that determine its activity in the integrated system. Thus he set himself the task of studying the connections existing in the organism and the interrelations between cerebral and internal visceral connections of the body. More precisely, he formulated the task of the investigation of corticovisceral correlations in four points:

1. The determination of the functional connections of the cerebral cortex with the viscera
2. The study of the possibility of forming conditional reflexes in response to stimulations conveyed from the viscera
3. The relatedness of conditional reflexes of exteroceptive and interoceptive origin
4. The analysis of the patterns of the temporary connections (conditional reflexes) of the visceral organs and tissue processes

Bykov reported on the conditional reflex functioning of the kidneys and liver, respiratory apparatus, digestive tract, metabolism, thermoregulation, and so on. He furthered the understanding of the influence of the central nervous system in the development of somatic illnesses. In some conditions, the central nervous system merely perceives the pathologically affected activity and integrates the pathological mechanism into the system. In other instances, certain physical or chemical stimuli influence the brain centers, which induce pathological alterations in the visceral organs. The central nervous system again registers these pathological alterations and integrates them. As a third variation, a psychological stimulus becomes the conditional stimulus of the former physical or chemical stimulus, and at the beginning temporarily induces a pathological state that, if long lasting or if stimulated frequently, recurs and eventually becomes permanent. The former constitutes the functional, and the latter the organic, phase of visceral illness.

The first, functional neurogenic phase of the specific visceral pathology follows a pattern similar to the other neuroses. It is the result of a stimulus and organism interaction, in which the response is localized in a specific organ. In this the psychological origin can be revealed. In the second, "organic," phase the illness cannot be distinguished from other organic conditions of different etiology.

PSYCHOSES

Pavlov always maintained that he was a physiologist and not a clinician, and all those descriptions in which he gave an explanation of psychotic illnesses were based on what might be called "excursions" into the clinical field. He never considered that psychotic conditions could be fully understood on the basis of observed behavioral manifestations alone. Psychotic manifestations, Pavlov thought, have a well-defined neurophysiological basis, but there is also a specific etiological factor that is the actual cause of the illness. In other words, he believed that there is something more involved in the development of these conditions that can be explained by the interaction of biologically and environmentally conditioned patterns and the effect of an ultramaximal stimulus.

In his descriptions of schizophrenia, manic-depressive psychosis, and paranoia he was very brief and confined himself to analogies, which resembled, to him, the conditions he had observed in his animal experiments.

Schizophrenia

Various forms of schizophrenia were first described in the mid-nineteenth century. Conolly and Morel described what is today known as simple schizophrenia, the latter introducing the term "dementia praecox." At about the same time, Hecker described the hebephrenic and Kahlbaum the catatonic schizophrenic. It fell to Kraepelin, however, to bring together all these findings into one broad category, which he labeled "dementia praecox." He considered this psychosis to be predetermined by heredity and believed its outcome to be inevitable. He saw dementia praecox as an organic disease of the brain but could find no evidence of malfunctioning beyond the behavioral-psychiatric manifestations.

Meyer (1906), introducing an etiological concept, considered dementia praecox to be an illness of faulty habit formation resulting from faulty response patterns, and he labeled the disease "parergesia." A few years later, however, Bleuler (1911) published his famous book on the illness, calling it, for the first time, "schizophrenia." Bleuler did not put forward any hypothesis on the etiology of schizophrenia but considered the main aspect of the disease to be the splitting and inappropriate interaction of the different components of the personality. In his well-known text-book on psychiatry (1916) he stated that schizophrenia appears to be a disease entity in the narrower sense, which, similar to the organic dementias, has several subcategories. Since then the term "schizophrenia" has been used for a group of mental illnesses, with symptoms that interfere with cognition, affectivity, and adaptive behavior in a characteristic way, leading, in the majority of cases (if untreated), to personality disorganization.

Pavlov considered schizophrenic symptoms as the expression of a chronic mental state, which, to him, resembled the condition obtained by a long-lasting hypnotic state. His contention that such a hypnotic state might continue for years was supported by a case described by Janet. Janet's patient slept for a period of five years and emerged from his hypnotic state only at night, when the ordinary daytime stimulations were interrupted.

Pavlov, to justify his opinion, proceeded to analyze a great variety of schizophrenic symptoms. In the beginning he analyzed the symptoms of the different catatonic states, starting with catatonic stupor. He realized that patients in stupor fail to react to questions under normal, everyday circumstances. On the other hand, he found that if the circumstances were changed, if these same patients were questioned in a soft voice in extremely quiet surroundings, then their reaction was favorable. Pavlov found an analogy here with those phenomena which were to be seen frequently at the beginning of experimentally induced sleep in animals. He saw that in the so-called "paradoxical" phase the animal loses its reaction to a strong stimulus, while still reacting normally to a weak one. This he correlated with the actions of the catatonic schizophrenic in a state of stupor.

Pavlov interpreted another catatonic symptom, negativism, on the same basis. Patients presenting this symptom permanently act contrary to request, for example, they refuse to eat if food is offered. This phenomenon he believed to be similar to one that he had observed in his experimental animals. He believed it to be correlated with the ultraparadoxical phase (third stage) of hypnosis, in which the positive conditional stimulus results in a negative effect.

Many other schizophrenic symptoms similarly bear a striking resemblance to familiar phenomena in normal hypnotized subjects. Among these are stereotypy, echolalia, echopraxia, and catalepsy.

Pavlov saw other correlations besides those between catatonic stupor and the paradoxical phase and negativism and the ultraparadoxical phase. He pointed out that symptoms such as the "silly" behavior of the hebephrenic, or the symptom of unwarranted excitement, could also frequently be seen during the time of normal awakening or falling asleep. His interpretation of these phenomena was that, with the beginning of general inhibition of the cerebral cortex, the subcortex is freed from its customary cortical control, and the basic mechanism of positive induction, an excitatory chaotic condition, ensues in all its centers.

The basis of the schizophrenic's hypnotic state may be either a hereditary or an acquired weakness of the nervous system, according to Pavlov. In the absence of prenatal pathology he considered that when a pathologically weakened nervous system, after an overwhelming stimulation, enters into a state of fatigue, the symptoms of schizophrenia are manifestations of this fatigue, which is characterized by the different stages of sleep inhibition. Pressing further along this line, Pavlov considered these hypnosis-like states to be due to overwhelming, or ultramaximal, stimulation of a specifically weakened nervous system. Hence, chronic hypnosis, as Pavlov saw schizophrenia, is, on the one hand, pathological, since it deprives the patient of his normal activity and leads to actual symptom formation, while, on the other hand, it is protective, since it conserves the cortical cells against a threatening destruction subsequent to an overwhelming task. In other words, Pavlov saw schizophrenic symptoms as a protection against further disorganization. Since certain forms of illness, such as catatonia, result in a percentage of speedy recoveries, he felt justified in stating that while the defense of the chronic hypnotic state lasts, the inhibitory process continues, preventing further destruction of the central nervous system.

Pavlov's concept of schizophrenia was not an isolated attempt to find an analogy for schizophrenic symptoms in normal psychological functioning, such as sleep. Contemporary German psychiatry discussed extensively the *müdes Denken* (tired, sleepy thinking) of the schizophrenic as a prevailing characteristic. In schizophrenic psychosis Pavlov considered and referred to certain analogies with hypnotic states. He did not consider the condition to be experimentally inducible by behavioral tools. In other words, while in neurosis he saw a specific reaction, depending upon the organism's preconstellation to stress, in schizophrenia he plainly considered that the manifestations bear a resemblance to conditions in the hypnotic states. He saw schizophrenia as a definite pathological condition with a specific acquired or hereditary weakness of the nervous system.

Manic-Depressive Psychosis

Kraepelin introduced the term "manic-depressive insanity" (1891), using it to label the illness described by Falret (1854) as *la folie circulaire*. The illness, in which manic and depressive episodes alternate, had been known from the time of Aretaeus, who described subjects in whom melancholia was followed by hilarious joy, with a subsequent reversal of the order.

Pavlov used in his interpretation of manic-depressive psychosis the contemporary concepts of Kretschmer. Kretschmer, on the basis of physical and psychological characteristics, distinguished two basic personality types: the fat, jovial, outgoing pyknics and the thin, flat, introspective asthenics. He considered the asthenic type to be more susceptible to schizophrenia, and the pyknic type to manic-depressive psychosis. Pavlov connected the asthenic characteristics with his inhibitory type and the pyknic characteristics with his excitable type and concluded that, while schizophrenia is the illness of the inhibitory type, manic-depressive psychosis is the illness of the excitable type.

Pavlov developed his concepts of manic-depressive psychosis as follows: At first he described the manifestations that take place after castration. He found that the activity of the animals of the strong "excitable" type after castration becomes irregular and chaotic. The change is temporary, and thereafter—in a month or so—a "circularity" sets in. The behavior of the dog is chaotic for a while, then it becomes spontaneously "more orderly." The periodicity becomes more distinct as time passes, but also the periods of "better work" become more frequent and of longer duration. Later, Pavlov extended his concepts on "circularity" and thought that not solely castration but other stresses may also produce in the excitable animal disturbed nervous activity.

In these experiments he observed a regular fluctuation, in

which there was at first a prominent inhibitory activity dominance. This was manifested in a reduction of conditioning ability, occasionally even to the degree at which conditional reflex formation became altogether impossible. It was also noticeable that formerly established conditional reflexes worked at a lowered intensity. This state was followed by a return to normality, and the temporary normality was seen to be succeeded by another period of pathological overactivity, a state in which prominent excitatory activity prevailed and in which conditioning ability increased. In this state conditional reflexes were formed with ease and formerly established conditional reflexes worked with great intensity. In some of the experimental animals he noticed that the alternating periods of decreased and increased activity occurred without the intermediate period of normality.

Pavlov attributed these alternating periods to a pathological unbalance between the excitatory and the inhibitory processes. He believed that in these animals the excitatory or inhibitory processes failed to restrict each other in their operations, which led to the fact that each of them had to reach an extreme intensity before being replaced by the other. In other words, he believed that the basic pathology is the result of an impairment of paradoxical induction.

The law of paradoxical induction holds that the excitatory process induces an inhibitory process both horizontally and vertically in the nervous system, the reverse also being true. When paradoxical induction fails to function normally, the balanced control of functioning is lost and the nervous system has to reach extremes (as in manic-depressive psychosis) before giving place to the opposite process.

Pavlov never considered the simple hypomanic or depressive conditions by themselves to be part of the illness. He saw them as a weakening of the inhibitory or the excitatory processes, respectively, due to external causes (i.e., the changing of a dynamic stereotype, etc.). On the other hand, manic-depressive psychosis he considered to be a separate form of illness of the "excitable" type.

Paranoia

In Pavlov's time paranoia was seen as a mental illness with the prominence of a systematized delusional system of unknown origin and dark prognosis. The illness was clearly differentiated from conditions resulting from toxic agents, such as alcohol and infection (syphilis). A further differentiation was from paranoid schizophrenia, in which a delusional system may become clinically prominent but, even so, remains a secondary reaction to the basic symptoms in psychopathology. Although several other conditions were also described in which delusions were prominent, no clear, physiologically based psychopathological theory existed at that time regarding this condition.

Pavlov described his views on paranoia in an article entitled "Attempt at a Physiological Interpretation of Compulsive Neurosis and Paranoia," which was published in the Russian booklet *Latest Reports on Physiology and Pathology of Higher Nervous Activity* (1933) and was translated into English in the *Journal of Mental Science* (1934) and into French in *L'Encéphale* (1935). He developed his concepts of this condition during the following animal experiments.

Petrova attempted the transformation of a positive conditional stimulus into a negative one and of an inhibitory, negative, stimulus into a positive conditional stimulus. She succeeded with some of the animals of the exceptionally strong type, while with others the stimuli could not, or could only temporarily, be reversed. Pavlov thought the lack of transformation of conditional stimuli to be due to a change of the excitatory process, which became "more stable and less inclined to yield to the inhibitory process." He confirmed this hypothesis by reproducing this modified state of the excitatory process by the same stimulations. Thereafter, he administered the positive conditional stimulus several times without reinforcement. As a result, he found that the conditional reflex to this conditional stimulus was extinguished more slowly than to other positive conditional stimuli under the same conditions. For the pathological phenomenon present he considered several descriptive names (i.e., "stagnancy," "uncommon inertness," "intensified concentration," "extraordinary tonicity") but preferred to use the term "pathological" or "increased inertness of the excitatory process." Similarly pathologically increased inertness of excitation, as present in obsessive-compulsive neurosis and paranoia, is the pathophysiological basis of stereotypy, iteration, perseveration. But, while in the latter the increased inertness of excitation is in the motor areas of the cerebral cortex, in compulsive neurosis and in paranoia the pathological pathodynamic structures are in areas that are connected with sensations, feelings, and ideas.

The pathophysiology of paranoia was further elaborated by Pavlov in the experiments in which he used two antagonistically acting metronomes. When protective inhibition developed as a result of the conflicting stimuli, in a certain stage of this general hypnotic state or local inhibition in the region of the metronome's action, the positively acting metronome became negative and the negatively acting metronome resulted in a positive conditional reflex.

This ultraparadoxical hypnotic phase, together with an increased, pathological inertness of excitation of a specific cortical area, Pavlov considered to be the pathophysiological basis of paranoia.

Pavlov applied these pathophysiological views in the analysis of psychiatric patients. Kretschmer's female patient, a mature girl, had normal sexual desire for a man she loved, but individual, moral, and social considerations hindered her from gratification. This Pavlov thought of as a strong enough "clash of the nervous processes" to lead to a pathological increased inertness of excitation at the corresponding cerebral areas, which are those connected with the struggling feelings and ideas. The girl acquired an irresistible, obsessive idea that her face reflected her sexual urges, started to hide her face, and avoided going out. She thought everyone looked at her and that everyone spoke about the expression of her face. Shortly afterward, one of her girl friends told her that, in the Garden of Eden, Eve had talked to a serpent, who was a sexual seducer. The patient immediately developed the idea that she had a serpent (sexual seducer) in her. The formation of this delusion Pavlov interpreted in the following manner.

> The girl had a strong and constant idea of her sexual purity, considering it under certain conditions, morally and socially shameful to have sexual desire, even though suppressed and not in the least gratified. On the basis of the general protective inhibition (ultraparadoxical phase) in which state our patient found herself and which in weak nervous systems normally accompanies a difficult state, this idea was irresistibly physiologically transformed into its opposite (slightly disguised), into an idea even bordering on a sensation of having the sexual seducer in her body.

There was a trend in Pavlov's time toward minimizing the differences between delusion and obsessive ideas, between paranoia and obsessive-compulsive neurosis. Janet thought that "the delusion of persecution is closely related to obsessive ideas," Kretschmer could not find "any essential differences between delusions and obsessive ideas," and Mallet claimed that in "delusion and obsession the organic damage is of the same nature." On the other hand, Pavlov emphasized the fact that, besides all the similarities of the two conditions, there are certain definite distinguishing characteristics. While in obsessive–compulsive conditions the patient has some insight into the morbid nature of his pathological state, the paranoid patient does not have this critical attitude toward his illness. The second difference Pavlov mentioned was the chronic course and incurability of paranoia.

On a pathophysiological basis Pavlov saw the difference between paranoia and obsessive-compulsive states in the degree of intensity of the increased, pathological inertness of excitation. In paranoia, he assumed a considerably greater intensity of the inertness of excitation, which produces on the periphery (on the basis of the law of negative induction) strong, widespread inhibition, which excludes the influence of the rest of the cerebral cortex with the opposing ideas.

Pavlov did not fail to recognize that the obsessive-compulsive state is a neurosis that, as any other neurosis, is the outcome of a stress in the environment-organism interaction, with a specific preconstellation in the central nervous system. On the other hand, in paranoia he saw a specific form of illness, a psychosis, similar to schizophrenia and manic-depressive psychosis.

THERAPY OF PSYCHIATRIC ILLNESSES

The presence of a dualistic philosophy in psychiatry is reflected in its two principal streams of thought, the psychological and the organic. At the beginning of the twentieth century the therapeutic implications of these two schools were to be seen in the various approaches, such as persuasion, suggestion, hypnosis, on the one hand, and drug treatment with opiates, barbiturates, and bromides, on the other.

Dominating the contemporary psychoanalytical stream in Europe was Freud's classical approach, which utilized the technique of "free association." The analyst tried to interfere as little as possible with the patient's stream of thought, while attempting to evoke the crucial material in the patient's early development that was instrumental in formulating the conflict that led to the neurotic symptoms. Freud's was a revolutionary concept and was indeed the greatest single step forward toward the establishment of a modern scientific psychiatry. In early Freudian writings it was not the removal of the symptoms but the expression of the conflict, not the insightful recognition of the problem but the cathartic abreaction of its emotional concomitants, that was believed to be therapeutically valuable. Thus he used a systematic desensitization (extinction) procedure as the core of psychoanalytical treatment.

While Freud used clinical experience, Pavlov applied experimental findings, in the formulation of his therapeutic concepts. On the one hand, he viewed the various forms of neuroses as specific reactions of specific organisms, with specific temperaments, to non-specific stress, while, on the other hand, he saw the faulty conditioning patterns of the psychotic illness as the outcome of a definite pathology. Pavlov's therapeutic indications extended to drug treatment, therapeutic suggestion, and sleep. He was also very much aware of the organisms' "self-healing" tendencies, and, as he expressed it in his address to the Pirogov Surgical Society (1927), the "chief curative measures we apply are interruption of all experimentation." However, he admitted that "sometimes we have recourse to additional methods." He found that for dogs of the inhibitory type five or six months of rest is the best therapeutic measure, while for the other type he considered, in addition, bromides and calcium salts to be useful.

Pavlov measured drug effect in changes of conditional reflex behavior. He reported on one of his experimental animals that presented chaotic conditional reflexes when exposed to daily experimentation, but normal conditional reflex patterns if exposed only every third day. By the administration of bromides Pavlov was able to restore and retain normal conditional reflex activity during daily experiments. This work on the effect of bromides was further elaborated by Popov in humans. He found that bromides do not weaken the activity of the excitatory process but strengthen the activity of the inhibitory process that promotes restoration. Therefore, after bromide administration, together with the intensification of the inhibitory process, there is sometimes a simultaneous increase of the positive reflexes. Similarly, it was found that the initial excitation observed during the early phase of alcohol consumption is the result not of an intensified excitatory process but of weakened internal inhibition. The functional "weakening" at a later stage, on the other hand, is the result not of a true inhibition but of weakened excitation. Thus ethyl alcohol fundamentally differs from caffeine and amphetamines, which are stimulants of the excitatory process.

Pavlov's school, by these findings, draws a line not merely between the true and pseudo-stimulants but also between the true hypnotic effect (with a primary intensification of inhibition) and conditions induced by the weakening of the excitatory process (which are manifest in the different varieties of narcosis). Pavlov's school also laid emphasis on the variability of the reactions to different dosages of a drug by different animals and in the different stages of experimentation. It was found that, the stronger the nervous system, the greater must be the dosage of the drug administered to produce its characteristic effect. When the temporary "weakness" of a nervous system is the result of disease, this nervous system grows stronger during the time of the recovery. Therefore, in this period, until full recovery, the dose of the drug should not be decreased but, rather, increased.

Pavlov made his greatest contribution to psychiatric therapy with his concept of sleep treatment. Sleep therapy was not his invention, having been used already in Aesculapius' shrines and also by contemporary psychiatrists (Klaesi). Pavlov's major contribution lay in defining its main uses. He pointed out its value in neuroses in protecting the central nervous system, by protective inhibition, from further disorganization. He also indicated sleep for those conditions in which the stimulus-response pattern has already been altered and in which a hypnotic state has already set in as a defense mechanism. Deepening of the hypnotic state he regarded as not only beneficial in the prevention of further stress but also as desirable in promoting the organism's self-protecting and reconstructing forces.

Prior to Pavlov, sleep therapy was almost exclusively used in conditions in which excitement dominated the clinical picture. These conditions required a relatively high dosage, close to the toxic of medication. Thus, Pavlov's indication of sleep therapy was the opposite of his predecessors and allowed him to use the drug in a relatively low dosage.

Sleep therapy was supervised by Petrova in the psychiatric clinic attached to Pavlov's laboratories. All possible external excitatory stimuli were eliminated from the sleep room. Cloetta mixture was used to induce sleep, and as an aid Pavlov employed the inhibitory effect of monotone, rhythmic stimuli (a slowly blinking blue light and a metronome beat). During the six to twelve days' sleeping period, patients were attended by a psychotherapist, whose role was to calm the wakeful patient by words that act directly on the second signal system.

In certain cases psychotherapy was also employed following sleep treatment. But while, in the former, psychotherapy served to reduce excitation and prepare the way for irradiating protective inhibition, in the latter it was used to stimulate the excitatory process and to bring the basic processes back to balance.

Special attention was paid by Pavlov to therapeutic suggestions. Since he considered words as signals that are connected with all the external and internal stimuli of the world, he assumed that they may signal all the stimuli and may evoke all the actions and reactions of the organism, which other stimuli condition. Therefore Pavlov considered suggestion as a simple but powerful conditional reflex. He stated that

> the word of the hypnotist to the hypnotised who is concentrating in a definite narrow region, evokes naturally deep external inhibition throughout the remaining mass of the hemispheres. This excludes all competing influence of all the other present and old traces of stimulation. Hence, the great, almost irresistible power of suggestion.

Pavlov limited therapeutic suggestion to specific indications. He restricted its administration to pathological conditions in which, because of the weakness of the second signal system, the first signal system is dominant, for example, hysteria or catatonic stupor. Under these circumstances he thought the suggested words (secondary or verbal signals) are directly transferred without any further elaboration into action.

Besides these specific therapeutic procedures, one of the greatest assets in Pavlov's therapeutic concepts was expressed by him in the following sentences:

> Though enormous progress has been made since olden times up to our day in the treatment of the mentally ill, still, I think, something remains to be desired in this respect. To keep patients still possessing a certain degree of self-consciousness, together with other, irresponsible patients, who may subject them on

the one hand, to strong stimulations in the form of screams and extraordinary scenes, and, on the other, to direct violence in most cases means creating conditions which to a still greater extent enfeeble the already weak cortical cells. Moreover, the violation of the patient's human rights, of which he is already conscious and which partly consists in restriction of his freedom, and partly in the fact that the attendants and medical personnel naturally and almost inevitably regard him as an irresponsible person, cannot but strike further heavy blows at the weak cortical cells. Consequently, it is necessary as quickly and as timely as possible to place such mentally diseased in the position of patients suffering from other illnesses which do not offend human dignity so manifestly.

Pavlovian psychiatry is discussed in detail in Pavlov's *Psychopathology and Psychiatry* compiled by Popov; in the second volume of the lectures on conditional reflexes translated and edited by Gantt; in Wells' book on Pavlov (*Toward a Scientific Psychology and Psychiatry*); and in Rokhlin's *Soviet Medicine in the Fight against Mental Disease.*

PART THREE

From Animal Experiments to Human Test Procedures

7

CONDITIONING

TECHNIQUES

IN PSYCHIATRY, as in other fields of medicine, the beginning of clinical science is the collection of observable data and the study of their interrelational patterns. The second step is methodical observation, utilizing specific means to extend and focus the scope of the observation in the experiment. Further development brings out the neurophysiological and neurochemical basis of psychiatry. Nevertheless, none of this information is necessarily etiological, for, even if the pathomechanism is revealed, the pathogenesis may remain hidden.

The different conditioning techniques are specific means that enable us to add further, qualitatively different observations to enlarge our understanding of psychiatric conditions. Since these techniques originate from the conditioning method, they reveal changes in conditional reflex functioning in the specific areas, which may indicate functional alterations in the central nervous system.

The conditional reflex is a physiological activity. The route of transmission from the afferent pathways of the conditional stimulus to the efferent pathways of the unconditional reflex has not yet been defined.

Since conditional reflexes are built on unconditional reflexes "written on by experience," an ontogenetic classification of these reflexes was offered by Angyan (intrauterine, newborn, child, and adult conditional reflexes). According to Angyan, the mature adult has developed most of his conditional reflexes to the utmost of his capability.

Hilgard and Marquis differentiated between conditioning techniques on the basis of the character of the conditional response. The members of the first group are primarily under the influence of the autonomic nervous system; those of the second group are primarily under the control of the central nervous system but are only semivoluntary; the members of the third group are completely voluntary.

A further general subdivision between the different conditioning techniques is based on Pavlov's brain model. In this model three levels of hierarchy are distinctly represented by the unconditional reflex and the conditional reflexes of primary and secondary (speech) order.

On this basis, conditioning techniques can be separated into those which provide information on the first signal system and those which provide information on the second signal system. In addition, there are techniques for studying the transmission from the first to the second signal system.

For clinical purposes, a comprehensive conditional reflex study using the different methods would include the autonomic techniques (GSR, plethysmography, salivary secretion, etc.), combined with the semivoluntary (eyelid closure, respiration, etc.) and voluntary (finger withdrawal, etc.) techniques, supplemented with Ivanov-Smolensky's procedure (conditional motor reflex with verbal reinforcement) and with a word association test.

In most psychiatric illnesses it is difficult to obtain full co-operation from the patient for a long time. The conditional reflex test, therefore, must be limited to a specific short procedure. Since many behavioral, psychological, and conditional reflex correlations are known, the test should be restricted to the specific manifestation under investigation.

CONDITIONING TECHNIQUES IN THE STUDY OF FIRST SIGNAL SYSTEM FUNCTIONS

The GSR Technique

One of the most widely used conditioning techniques employs galvanic skin resistance (GSR) as a measuring device.

The GSR commonly denotes the amount of resistance (conductance) change produced by the electricity elicited by the chemical action of sweat gland secretion. Sweat gland activity is directly influenced by the autonomic nervous system.

The term "autonomic" has been the subject of controversy for many years, since the system it describes is morphologically connected with and functionally controlled by the central nervous system and therefore is not really independent. For example, in the GSR, emotional relations (psychogalvanic response [PGR]) are strongly reflected.

The GSR has been widely used in laboratories, although its physiological basis is not yet fully understood. Sweat glands are innervated by the sympathetic fibers of the autonomic nervous system, yet their behavior toward drugs is somewhat similar to what their action would be if innervated by parasympathetic fibers. For example, they remain unaffected by adrenalin, are stimulated by pilocarpine, and are inhibited by atropine (Best and Taylor).

These facts were graphically demonstrated in Dale's and Feldberg's animal experiments, in which excitation of the sympathetic fibers to the foot pads of the cat resulted in sweating and the appearance of acetylcholine in the eserinized fluid perfusing the paw.

The basic techniques for measuring the GSR were developed independently by Ferré and Tarchanoff. At present, several variations exist, but, in general, those in use are monopolar or bipolar techniques.

For the instrumentation, the subject is seated in a soundproofed, temperature and humidity-controlled room. An active silver electrode is attached to the palm of the hand, and the reference electrodes are placed midway between his wrist and elbow.

The principal instrument is a Wheatstone bridge. The subject's skin resistance is balanced to the closest approximation across the bridge by a decade resistance unit. The remaining unbalanced portion is supplied by means of a D.C. amplifier, which drives the galvanometer of a chart recorder.

In the conditioning procedure, an indifferent conditional

stimulus is associated with a specific unconditional stimulus. After several associated administrations, the formerly indifferent stimulus is tried alone, and, if conditioned, it results in a skin resistance decrease. An electroshock to the finger tip is most commonly used as the unconditional stimulus, but some investigators prefer a strong tone. Any sensory organ can be used for the conditional stimulus (Bass and Hull, tactile; Hovland, auditory; White, Schlosberg, and Keller, visual).

In the evaluation of the GSR the subject's basal resistance is established. The response to the unconditional stimulus is measured. The time lapse between the stimulus administered and the starting of the response (and also the recovery time when the change due to the stimulus is over) are registered. The frequency of the subject's response to the conditional stimulus, if administered alone or in combination preceding the effect of the unconditional stimulus, is expressed by frequency analysis, whereas amplitude analysis deals with the quantity intensity of skin resistance change to the different stimuli.

GSR conditioning presents several problems, both theoretical and practical. One is the problem of the stimuli—conditional stimulus and unconditional stimulus—to be used. The commonly used electroshock is not a real unconditional stimulus of the GSR function. Habituation of the shock creates problems in the experimental procedure. This uncertainty regarding the unconditional stimulus and the conditional stimulus is even more evident when an auditory stimulus is used by some as a conditional stimulus and by others as an unconditional stimulus. There are wide individual variations in the GSR even in the normal population, and similarly among patients, presenting similar psychopathology. Furthermore, besides the interindividual variations, there are also intraindividual variations, that is, the same subject on consecutive days or even on the same day may present different readings. There is, furthermore, a change (drop) in the resistance to any external stimulation (orienting reflex). But there is also a GSR change to intensive thinking (problem solving or emotionally loaded experiences). However, that the psychologically meaningful stimulus would have a greater effect for the GSR than an indifferent physical stimulus could not be proved.

Plethysmography

In 1863 Philipeaux and Vulpian made the observation that after section and subsequent degeneration of the twelfth (hypoglossus) cranial nerve, stimulation of the chorda tympani going to the tongue caused a slow and prolonged contraction of the lingual muscles together with vasodilation. Similar observations in other areas were made by Sherrington and Rogowitz. The same effect can be obtained by acetylcholine. The effect can be intensified by eserine but cannot be counteracted by atropine, meaning that peripheral vasodilatation is not clearly a parasympathetic effect. Vasomotor reactions are regulated by hypothalamic centers, and several theories have been suggested.

The plethysmograph is an instrument that was designed to measure changes in the volume of the limb caused by alterations in the amount of blood circulating in the vessels. The measured limb was suspended in water that almost filled a cylindrical chamber. The recording was done through the changes in air pressure transmitted by water pressure onto a meter that registered on a kymograph. The air-pressure change originated from the varying size of the limb transmitted to the water and air in the closed cylindrical chamber. This clinical instrument was invented by Piegu and later modified by Lehmann. At the present, Shmavonian's finger plethysmograph is the one most generally used. It is based on a thermo–battery, that is, instead of measuring volume changes (due to vasodilatation or vasoconstriction), it measures changes of illumination.

The procedure is conducted in a soundproof, temperature and humidity-controlled room, in which the subject sits in a comfortable, relaxed position. He is asked not to make any deliberate movement, and involuntary movements are minimized by placing the instrument in a fixed position on the arm of a chair.

Conditioning follows the same pattern as used with other techniques. An adequate unconditional stimulus is preceded by an inadequate stimulus. After several combined associated presentations of the two stimuli the inadequate stimulus becomes conditioned, that is, conditionally sufficient to elicit the formerly specific response to the unconditional adequate stimulation. Traugott considers pain and cold to be components of the unconditional defensive reflex and thus not extinguishable by repetition. Similarly, these two stimuli appear to be adequate for unconditional stimulation to obtain vasoconstriction. In humans, an electroshock to the finger tip or thermal stimuli is used. Notwithstanding theoretical considerations regarding pain, the electrical stimulus habituates quickly. The administration of the thermal stimulus presents technical difficulties. Astrup touched the free forearm with a metal container filled with ice; Lilly used a container of warm water; Rogov passed water through a coil fixed to one of the subject's arms. Others (Prescott, etc.) used an auditory (strong sound) as the unconditional stimulus.

The conditional stimulus may arrive through any sensory organ. However, auditory (Astrup, Rogov, Pshonik, etc.) and visual (Prescott, Rogov, etc.) stimuli are the most widely used.

The evaluation of the results follows the same lines as in the GSR technique. When the response has subsided, frequency and amplitude of the responses to the unconditional, combined, and conditioned stimuli are measured, together with the reaction (delay between the beginnings of stimulus and response) and the recovery time. Some recommend starting from a zero plethysmogram (Pshonik), on which the curve of pulse waves is almost horizontal. Since such ideal conditions cannot be obtained until after approximately thirty preliminary sessions, in psychiatric work this is omitted.

The pioneer of the plethysmographic technique in conditioning was Tsitovitch (1918), who demonstrated that in humans a tone, given simultaneously with cooling, after approximately twenty-five associated-combined administrations, leads to the same plethysmographic change as the actual temperature. Systematic studies were initiated which revealed that the first signs of the conditional reflex appear after approximately the fifth trial, while 70–90 associated administrations are needed for the full establishment of the conditional reflex (Bykov).

A technical advance, polygraphic instrumentation, made it possible to have simultaneous recordings of several conditioning aspects of the organism. Simultaneous recording of GSR and plethysmograph is favored by several investigators. It should be noted that the number of stimuli required to extinguish the orienting reflex is higher for the GSR and that the number of associated stimulations required to establish a conditional reflex is higher for the plethysmograph. Thus, extreme care is necessary in devising the programming and in analyzing the data for interpretation.

Defensive Finger Withdrawal

Finger withdrawal is a conscious, willed action with a center located in the precentral area of the frontal lobe. That finger withdrawal can be directly observed is a great advantage over the GSR and plethysmography.

The finger withdrawal technique derives, in principle, from Bekhterev and was introduced by Protopopov (1909). A mild electric shock to the finger tip is used as the unconditional stimulus. The finger is withdrawn as a defense to the pain, hence it is called the "defensive reflex." The impulse from the pain stimulus travels from the specifically developed receptors, by way of the spinothalamic fibers, to the thalamus. Here it is perceived as pain. However, the place of its origin is located in the post central parietal area of the cerebral cortex. The reflex circuit closes in the frontal cortical function of finger withdrawal.

In this technique, only electric shock is used as the unconditional stimulus, while the conditional stimulus may arrive through any sensory organ. Auditory stimuli are the most frequently used. The technique is carried out in a conditioning chamber adjoining the experimenter's room. Here the subject is seated, and his index finger is placed on the electrodes of the unconditional stimulus apparatus. Astrup connected the index finger by a cord to the vertical writer of a kymograph. Gantt took muscle potential records (E.M.G.), while Humphrey used a modified Watson apparatus that indicated by a light system whether the subject's index finger remained in position or moved.

The subject is previously informed that his reaction to an electric current will be measured and that he may take his finger off if he feels the current. The strength of the current used is above the pain threshold of the subject. The conditional stimulus is administered on a number of occasions. Then the unconditional stimulus is administered alone, and afterward the paired associations, in which the conditional stimulus precedes the unconditional stimulus. The accuracy of the evaluation depends on the instrumentation.

With Humphrey's method only the occurrence of the response can be registered; with Astrup's method the actual degree of the response can be measured; and this can be done even more precisely by Gantt's method. The finger withdrawal technique is simple to perform but needs the subject's co-operation. The technique's greatest disadvantage is that it deals with a function that can be influenced by will.

Defensive Eyelid Closure

Blinking is a semivoluntary activity. One blinks automatically; on the other hand, blinking can also be regulated by will. Eyelid closure is the activity of the seventh nerve (facialis), whose function can be altered by central (nuclear, supranuclear) or peripheral nerve pathology. The pioneering work in eyelid closure conditioning was done by Cason, whose early experiments were continued by many investigators (Miller, Gantt, Varga, Franks, etc.).

The unconditional stimulus in this technique is a puff of air directed to the cornea. This air pressure affects the trigeminal (fifth nerve) receptors. The unconditional reflex circuit ends in a facial (seventh nerve) activity, in blinking. A few investigators used a mild electric shock administered to the cheek as an unconditional stimulus. The conditional stimulus may arrive through any sensory organ. Auditory conditional stimuli are the most widely used. In the conditioning procedure the subject sits comfortably in an armchair in the conditioning chamber. An air puff pipe is placed close to the cornea, and the unconditional stimulus is administered through it. The conditional stimulus is received through earphones. The eyelid closure blinking response was transmitted to a kymograph in the classical experiments (in which two Grass electrodes are fixed above and below the eye). More recently, a photoelectric cell has been used.

Responses to the unconditional stimulus, to the conditional stimulus, and to their associations are registered and evaluated. The frequency of both adequate and inadequate responses gives information on the conditional reflex functions of this specific area. Amplitude of the responses is the measure of their strength. While the eyelid closure technique is one of the simplest of the conditioning procedures and provides valid information about a physiological function that can be influenced by will, its great disadvantage lies in the great variability between subjects in frequency and strength of blinking. Many subjects cannot be tested because of their extreme blinking frequency; a few others fail because of corneal hyper- or hyposensitivity.

Other Techniques
1. Central Nervous System: Electroencephalography
Physiology: The dominant wave of the normal electroencephalogram is the occipital alpha rhythm. This appears as an 8–12 per second frequency.

History: Loomis, Harvey, and Hobart (1936) noted that a previously indifferent tone, coinciding or preceding an unconditional light stimulus administered several times in succession, blocked the occipital alpha rhythm. Thus, the tone—here conditional stimulus—took on the role of the light—here unconditional stimulus. They also noted that this alpha block response to the tone was extinguishable. They found the alpha block to the tone to be extinguished after permanently withholding the light stimulus (reinforcement). This technique was further elaborated by Travis and Egan, Knott and Henry, Jasper and Cruikshank, and others.

The unconditional stimulus: The unconditional stimulus for this technique is a visual (light) stimulus that depresses the occipital alpha rhythm on the electroencephalogram.

The conditional stimulus: An auditory (sound) stimulus is used as conditional stimulus in this technique.

Procedure: The subject is asked to lie down comfortably in a dark, soundproofed room adjoining that in which the instruments are kept. The electrodes are placed on the occipital cortical area of the skull and on the right ear. The procedure begins with the administration of several consecutive light signals alone and sound signals alone, to ascertain the response to the unconditional stimulus and also to extinguish the orienting reflex. Trials with the sound alone follow the combined conditioning trials. The conditional reflex is considered established when at least two consecutive adequate responses to the conditional stimulus alone occur. The criteria of an adequate response is a block of the occipital alpha rhythm on the record.

Remarks: This technique is rarely used because it needs the full co-operation of the patient. Subjects with an insufficient response to the unconditional stimulus are common.

2. *Autonomic Nervous System: The Pupillary Reflex*

Physiology: The pupils are innervated by fibers of the autonomic nervous system. Direct stimulation of the sympathetic fibers produces a dilatation in which pupils are described as mydriatic. Direct stimulation of the parasympathetic fibers produces a constriction in which the pupils are described as myotic. The same myotic reaction occurs if the sympathetic innervation is cut off.

History: Cason was the first to use the pupillary reflex in human conditioning procedures.

The unconditional stimulus: The unconditional stimulus for this technique is a visual (light) stimulus that constricts the pupils.

The conditional stimulus: The conditional stimulus used in this technique is an auditory (bell) stimulus.

Procedure: The subject is comfortably seated in a dark, soundproof room and asked to keep his eyes on a light source within the apparatus (Hudgins, Weller, and Cason). A telescope directs the light into the observer's eye, and the diameter of the pupil is measured on a millimeter scale. More recently, photometric techniques have been elaborated (Zubin).

The procedure begins with the administration of light signals alone and sound signals alone to ascertain the response to the unconditional stimulus and also to extinguish the orienting reflex. Trials with the sound alone follow the combined conditioning trials. The conditional reflex was considered established when at least two consecutive adequate responses to the conditional stimulus alone occurred. The criteria of an adequate response was a pupillary constriction on the record.

Evaluation: The responses are measured (metrically) on the record.

Remarks: It needs full co-operation from the patient. Tatarenko finds it an extremely sensitive indicator of psychopathology.

3. *Autonomic Nervous System: Salivary Secretion*

Physiology: The three main salivary glands, the parotid, submaxillary, and sublingualis are innervated by autonomic fibers of the seventh and ninth cranial nerves (facialis and glossopharyngeus). Parasympathetic drugs (hyosciamine, atropine, belladonna) reduce salivary secretion.

History: The first experiments on humans were carried out by Kleitman and Crisler (1927) with the application of this technique.

The Unconditional Stimulus: The unconditional stimulus for this technique is food that produces salivary secretion (lollipop, sweetened lemon juice, etc.).

The Conditional Stimulus: Any formerly indifferent stimulus through any sensory organs can be used; however, in actual experiments auditory stimuli (tone, sound) are usually given preference.

Procedure: A cotton roll is inserted under the tongue, or parotid capsules are placed over the buccal orificium of the salivary glands. The association of stimuli (conditional and unconditional—in that order) must be conducted on consecutive days or on the same day with different time intervals before eating. The conditional reflex was considered established when at least two consecutive adequate responses to the conditional stimulus occurred. The criteria of an adequate response was a definite increase of salivary secretion.

Evaluation: The dental cotton roll (or parotid capsules) is weighed.

Remarks: Chemically, the saliva secreted to the conditional stimulus and not to the unconditional stimulus is closer to the spontaneously secreted saliva; the amylase activity of the saliva secreted to the conditional stimulus is greater than that to the unconditional stimulus. Depression reduces salivary secretion similarly to the parasympatholytic drugs.

4. *Peripheral Nervous System: The Patellar Reflex*

Physiology: The patellar reflex is elicited by a blow with a reflex hammer on the tendon of the quadriceps muscle. This afferent stimulus is transmitted through the upper lumbar spinal region to the efferent nerve and results in an extension of the lower extremity. Administration of the conditional stimulus and the unconditional stimulus alone is followed by the combined conditioning trials. The conditional reflex was considered established when at least two consecutive adequate responses to the conditional stimulus alone occurred.

History The conditioning of the patellar reflex dates back to Shewaler (1926).

The Unconditional Stimulus. The unconditional stimulus for this technique is a blow applied with a reflex hammer at the specified point below the knee.

The Conditional Stimulus: The conditional stimulus, although it may be administered through any sensory organ, is most frequently auditory (a bell).

Procedure: The subject sits comfortably in a chair. A light harness is adjusted to his leg. The harness carries an arm that shows, over a graduated quadrant, the intensity (height) of each response. At first, the conditional stimulus and the unconditional stimulus are presented alone, then in association, in which the bell precedes the blow. Finally, the responses to the conditional stimulus alone are taken. The conditional reflex is considered established when at least two consecutive adequate responses to the conditional stimulus occur. The criteria of an adequate response is a patellar reflex.

Evaluation: The height of each response is measured metrically.

Remarks: Pfaffmann needed approximately two hundred combined presentations (conditional stimulus and unconditional stimulus) before he succeeded in eliciting the response to the conditional stimulus alone.

5. *Mixed Functions: Respiration*

Physiology: Respiration is regulated by the medullary respiratory centers but can also be influenced voluntarily.

History: Since the studies of Garvey (1933), a great number of investigators have used this technique (Voitkevich, Reese, Golubykh, Gubler, Boronkova, Konradi, Bebeshinas, and others).

The Unconditional Stimulus: Garvey used faradic stimulation, Boronkova used ammonia gas inhalation, while Bebeshinas used a mixture of carbon dioxide and air. Frequency increase and irregularity, intensification, and interrupted respiration were the responses, respectively.

The Conditional Stimulus: Voitkevich pointed out that any indifferent stimulus can become a conditional signal for the specific unconditional respiratory change if, in consecutive administrations, it precedes the unconditional stimulus. Auditory (buzzer, metronome beat) or vibratory stimuli are most frequently used.

Procedure: A rubber cord is applied around the chest at the level of the nipples.

Evaluation: Respiration is measured in pressure and air-volume changes.

Remarks: The recording of respiration during other conditioning procedures has increased since the introduction of modern polygraphs.

6. *Other Functions:*

In human development, the various conditional reflexes extend during development. The newborn baby functions almost entirely by unconditional reflexes. He empties his bladder or bowel as a result of pressure and even breathes to the unconditional stimulus of oxygen lack and carbon dioxide pressure. Other functions are also unconditionally regulated; for instance, the sexual functioning of many animals is mainly dominated by the unconditional direction of endocrine hormones.

As time passes and conditioning goes on, eating and sleeping habits develop. Time conditioning is one of the most important achievements that permit a subtle control over various functioning. The child, on reaching a certain age, no longer eats or sleeps only because he is hungry or sleepy but becomes hungry or sleepy at certain time intervals. The same applies to the sexual function, which is not activated solely by hormones but also by stimulation through other organs, for example, touch, smell, etc., or even words, talking, reading, or merely by thinking of sex.

Several of the conditional reflex functions that contribute to resistance have been described. The conditioned increase of the white blood cell count was described by Urin and Zenkevich; conditioned blood clotting by Marakovsky; immunological reactions, etc., by Doroshvich, Dolin, Krylov, and others; urinary secretion by Fuller and others.

Thus, conditioning studies opened a new pathway to the study of organic and metabolic pathology.

CONDITIONING TECHNIQUES IN STUDY OF TRANSMISSION
FROM FIRST TO SECOND SIGNAL SYSTEM

First technique: The autonomic pupillary reflex technique is used. The regular procedure applied in conditioning is followed (i.e., the unconditional pupillary constriction to light and to an auditory conditional stimulus).

The subject is asked to squeeze a dynamometer at a command. This closes the bell-light circuit. When pupillary constriction becomes conditioned to the bell, the unconditional light stimulus is omitted. When the verbal command (secondary conditional stimulus) results in the reflex, the conditional stimulus (bell) is also omitted. Transmission from the unconditional reflex system to the conditional reflex system (pupillary constriction from light to bell) and from the first to the second signal system (pupillary constriction from bell to verbal command) can thus be studied.

Second technique: Ivanov–Smolensky's technique is used. The procedure is as follows. The subject places his index finger on a telegraph key. Then an auditory conditional stimulus (a bell signal) is administered, which is followed by the verbal command "Press." When the subject presses spontaneously after the bell signal, the conditional motor reflex is established and the command "Press" is omitted. Then the conditional stimulus is replaced by the corresponding verbal signal (it rings). When this signal results in the reflex, the conditional stimulus is also omitted. Transmission from the unconditional reflex system to the conditional reflex system (motor activity from a verbal command to a bell) and from the first to the second signal system (motor activity from a bell to the corresponding verbal signal) can thus be studied.

CONDITIONING TECHNIQUES IN THE STUDY OF THE SECOND
SIGNAL SYSTEM

Verbal signals are secondary conditional stimuli. The basic difference between verbal signals and this secondary conditional stimuli is that at birth there is no reflex response to any verbal signal, but only to their auditory elements. The process by which the human child develops these verbal signals as meaningful conditional stimuli is physiological in nature.

The development of verbal signals follows the same pattern as that of other conditional stimuli. At first, several words could elicit the same or a similar response (conditional stimulus generalization), while by further elaboration—differentiation—only a specific word will elicit it. Thus increasingly specific, concrete, and, later, abstract ideas can be reflected by a single word.

The response to the unconditional or primary conditional stimuli is always skeletomuscular or visceral, but the response to verbal stimuli may remain on a verbal level. These secondary verbal signals enrich human life by abstractions that lead to communication (and insight) and also to the possibility of consciously influencing activities.

The four most widely used techniques applied in the study of the second signal system are described as follows.

First technique: The autonomic pupillary constriction is conditioned to a heteroverbal-secondary conditional stimulus, as described before. Then the command "Contract" is given by the subject himself, at first loudly, later as a whisper, and finally subvocally. The pupillary light reaction, which is conditioned at first to a bell (auditory conditional stimulus) and afterward to the command "Contract" (heteroverbal conditional stimulus), finally responds to the subject's own command (autoverbal conditional stimulus, or will). The technique provides valid information on the possible voluntary influence of autonomic functioning.

Second technique: Ivanov-Smolensky's technique is used. The subject is asked to press a rubber balloon at command. Then, prior to the verbal command, colored lights in consecutive flashes of red, green, and yellow are presented. Finally, their written symbols are projected. Under physiological conditions, the voluntary action of pressing a rubber balloon becomes conditioned to visual stimuli, then to their corresponding verbal stimuli, and finally to the written symbols of the verbal stimuli.

Third technique: Krasner described a collection of techniques in use for the conditioning of verbal behavior. The sentence-completion technique is the most widely used (Taffel, Cohen, etc.).

This technique is based on the reinforcement of sentences starting with a specific pronoun or by reinforcing sentences with a specific group of verbs. A verb in the past tense is written on the center of the index card, and below the verb six random pronouns are written. Subjects are asked to form complete sentences, using verbs in the center and starting with one of the pronouns. Of the six pronouns only one was reinforced. As non-verbal reinforcing cues, visual (flashing lights) or auditory (buzzer or bell) stimuli were used. Among the verbal cues, one of the following was applied: "mmm-hmm," "uhha," "yeah," "good," "right," "fine," "I see."

Fourth technique: The technique of studying "word associations," was introduced in the late nineteenth century by Galton. Word-association tests described in the literature vary greatly in technical details, and even more so in interpretation. It is interesting to note that the Freudian and Pavlovian schools both used them.

The Pavlovian school uses free association for gaining more detailed and accurate information on the effect of the psychopathological process. While for the Freudian school free association reveals information on the dynamics of the individual, for Pavlovians the same technique indicates the extensiveness and intensity of psychopathology.

Ivanov-Smolensky was among the first to think that this technique might reveal information on second signal system activity. Since then it has been applied in studies on the ontogenetic development of the second signal system by Krasnogorski and Luria and in an extensive conditional reflex study on schizophrenia by Astrup.

In the following chapter the different test procedures developed by the application of these techniques will be discussed.

8

DIAGNOSTIC TEST
PROCEDURES

DIAGNOSTIC TESTS, based on conditional reflex phenomena, for psychiatric purposes are partly replicas of Pavlov's behavioral animal experiments in humans. Other procedures reveal information on the transmission from the first to the second signal system and/or second signal system functions.

The following functions are tested.

FIRST SIGNAL SYSTEM

1. *Unconditional reflex functioning:* This test is based on the first experiment described in chapter 2 "Behavioral Observations," in which a dog was fed by placing food in its mouth in close connection with the sensory end organs. The secretion observed was called an unconditional reflex. These reflexes were described as purely conducting and were assumed to be congenital and not capable of modification through training or education. They follow the patterns that Sherrington revealed as characteristics of the the spinal cord reflexes. Applied to humans, voluntary, semivoluntary, and autonomic techniques are used (i.e., finger withdrawal to an electric shock, eyelid closure to an air puff to the cornea, decrease in skin resistance to a strong tone, etc.).

The strength and the duration of the unconditional reflex are measured to different intensities of stimuli, as is the time lapse—latency—between stimulus and response.

2. *Orienting reflex functioning:* This test is based on the

seventh experiment described in chapter 2, in which a conditional food reflex was established to a metronome beat. When an unknown strong sound was suddenly introduced, the dog moved in the direction of the new sound and did not respond to the conditional stimulus. This startle reaction was called an "orienting reflex." This concept was further elaborated after the advent of the electroencephalograph. In Gastaut's hypothesis the application of a stimulus at the beginning of any conditioning procedure results in generalized cortical desynchronization (startle response), which is followed by a desynchronization in the specific cortical area (orienting response). The startle response is conceived as the result of the stimulation of brain stem reticular formation activity; the orienting response as the result of the stimulation of thalamic reticular formation activity.

The startle response can be measured by simultaneous recording of voluntary, semivoluntary, and autonomic reflexes. It is manifested in the simultaneous responses in the different systems to the non-specific stimulation (i.e., finger withdrawal, eyelid closure, decrease of skin resistance, etc.). Similarly, the orienting response is a reflex to the non-specific stimulation, but in a specific area (i.e., finger withdrawal to a tone, eyelid closure to a metronome beat, decrease of skin resistance to a red light, etc.). While the extinction rate of the startle response is expressed in the number of reflexes in several areas, that of the orienting response is confined to the number of reflexes in the specific area. Latency time between stimulus and response and both the strength and the duration of the latter are registered.

3. *Conditional reflex functioning:* Conditional reflex formation is described in the second and third experiments in chapter 2. In puppies fed on milk merely the sight of the milk alone resulted in salivary secretion. Similarly, if a metronome beat was made to precede feeding, after several repetitions salivation began in response to the metronome alone. As seen from these experiments, the consistent temporal association of the conditional and unconditional stimuli, in that order, is the prerequisite for conditional reflex formation. Pavlov

believed the conditional reflex to be a cerebral-cortical function. This supposition has been discarded by some of his successors, and there is also some experimental evidence suggesting that the conditional reflex can be formed in decorticated animals in the subcortical structures.

In human conditioning tests, a formerly indifferent stimulus to a specific activity is developed, under the conditions, into a specific stimulus for the specific function. Voluntary, semivoluntary, and autonomic techniques are used, that is, finger withdrawal to an electric shock to the tip of the finger is conditioned to a white light; eyelid closure to a puff of air on the cornea is conditioned to a metronome beat; decrease of skin resistance to a strong tone is conditioned to a red light; and so on. During the conditioning procedure the originally indifferent stimulus for the function precedes the unconditional stimulus on consecutive occasions. The number of associated (conditional and unconditional) stimulations required before the reflex response to the conditional stimulus alone is established is the measure of conditioning ability.

Latency time between stimulus and response and also the strength and the duration of the latter are recorded. The extinction of the startle and the orienting reflexes is the prerequisite for this procedure.

4. *Delayed reflex functioning:* Delayed reflex formation is described in the fourth experiment in chapter 2, in which a conditional food reflex was established to a metronome beat; thereafter, the length of the conditional stimulation was considerably increased. The postponed conditional reflex from the origin to the end of the prolonged stimulus is described by Pavlov as delayed reflex, which he conceived to be the result of the inhibitory process (internal inhibition). Delayed reflex formation is assumed to be a cerebral-cortical function. The number of combined presentations of the prolonged conditional stimulus (with the unconditional stimulus) before the postponement of the response is the measure of delayed reflex formation. Latency time between stimulus and response and also the strength and the duration of the latter are recorded. Delayed reflex formation can be tested by voluntary, semi-

voluntary, and autonomic techniques. Extinction of the startle and orienting responses and conditional reflex formation are the prerequisites for this procedure.

5. *Trace reflex functioning:* Trace reflex formation is described in the fifth experiment in chapter 2, in which metronome beats (conditional stimulus) were presented before feeding (unconditional stimulus), with an interval between the two. Pavlov described a trace reflex as the conditional reflex with a prolonged time interval between the conditional stimulus and the unconditional stimulus. While in delayed reflexes the conditional stimulus is prolonged and the reflex postponed to the end of this elongated stimulus, in a trace reflex the conditional stimulus remains unaltered, but the reflex appears following a time interval after the conditional stimulus. Both are assumed to be cerebral-cortical functions. The number of associated stimulations with the time interval between conditional stimulus and unconditional stimulus, before the reflex is established, is the measure of trace reflex formation. The strength and the duration of the response are recorded. Trace reflex formation can be tested by voluntary, semivoluntary, and autonomic techniques. Extinction of the startle and orienting responses and conditional reflex formation are prerequisites for this procedure.

6. *Time conditioning:* This is a "late" trace reflex, as described in the sixth experiment in chapter 2, in which dogs were fed every thirty minutes until they salivated spontaneously at the same time intervals. In humans this phenomenon can be observed in the functioning of several organs or tested in an experimental situation by voluntary, semivoluntary, and autonomic techniques, administered at regular intervals. The number of stimulations with fixed intervals that are required before the establishment of the conditional reflex indicates conditioning ability to time.

7. *Extinction of the conditional reflex:* In the eighth experiment described in chapter 2 the established conditional food reflex to a metronome beat was not reinforced. During the course of the procedure the conditional stimulus became ineffective. Pavlov called this phenomenon "extinction" and con-

sidered it to be a type of internal inhibition that is a function of the cerebral cortex. In human tests the procedure follows the same lines as in the animal experiments. Voluntary, semi-voluntary, and autonomic techniques are used. The number of non-reinforced stimulations required before no response occurs to the previously conditioned conditional stimulus is the measure of this function. The time for developing extinction is directly proportional to the frequency of non-reinforced conditional stimuli. Extinction of the startle and orienting reflexes and conditional reflex formation are the prerequisites for this procedure.

8. *Conditional stimulus generalization:* The phenomenon whereby stimuli, quantitatively or qualitatively different from the conditional stimulus, temporarily result in a conditional reflex is called "generalization." Generalization was described in the thirteenth experiment in chapter 2, in which a conditional food reflex was established to a metronome beat of a certain frequency, and thereafter, temporarily, salivary secretion was observed to several other metronome-beat frequencies. In human tests the procedure follows the same lines as in the animal experiments. Voluntary, semivoluntary, and autonomic techniques are used. The total number of responses to the administered indifferent non-reinforced stimuli before differentiation (no response) takes place provides the measure of this function. Extinction of the startle and orienting reflexes and conditional reflex formation are the prerequisites for this procedure.

9. *Conditional stimulus differentiation:* The opposite to generalization was described in the fourteenth experiment in chapter 2, in which the conditional reflex to a certain specific metronome beat frequency became limited to this specific metronome-beat frequency and no longer responded to any other stimulus. Pavlov called this phenomenon "differentiation" and considered it a type of internal inhibition that is the function of the cerebral cortex. Although it was found that after removal of the neocortex a crude type of differentiation still remained, the cerebral cortex is assumed to be the morphological substrate of differentiation. In human tests

the procedure follows the same lines as in the animal experiments. Voluntary, semivoluntary, and autonomic techniques are used. The total number of reinforced and non-reinforced stimuli required before differentiation takes place is the measure of this function. Extinction of the startle and orienting reflexes, conditional reflex formation, and extinction of generalization are the prerequisites for this procedure.

10. *Secondary conditional reflex functioning:* This is described in the twenty-third experiment in chapter 2, in which the salivary secretion of the dog was conditioned to a metronome beat at first and thereafter to the presentation of a black rectangle that preceded the metronome beat. The conditional reflex to the black rectangle Pavlov called a "secondary conditional reflex," since it is secondary in order of formation to the metronome beat. The secondary conditional reflex is assumed to be a cerebral-cortical function. In human tests the same procedure is followed as in animal experiments; voluntary, semivoluntary, and autonomic techniques are used. The number of combined presentations of the secondary and primary conditional stimuli, in that order, before the conditional reflex develops to the secondary conditional stimulus alone is the measure of secondary conditional reflex formation. Extinction of the startle and orienting reflexes and conditional reflex formation are the prerequisites of this procedure.

11. *Mobility or reversal of conditional stimuli:* Mobility or reversal of conditional stimuli was described in the thirty-first experiment in chapter 2, in which two reflexes, a positive and a negative conditional food reflex, were established to the auditory stimuli of different metronome beat frequencies. Thereafter, the negative conditional stimulus was continuously associated with feeding, while the positive conditional stimulus was no longer reinforced. In some of the animals the reversal of the conditional stimuli was successful, while in others they were not transformable. The phenomenon of changing a positive conditional stimulus into a negative one and a negative conditional stimulus into a positive one was called by Pavlov "mobility" and was assumed to be a cerebral-cortical function. In human tests the same procedure is fol-

lowed as in animal experiments. Voluntary, semivoluntary, and autonomic techniques are used. The total number of stimuli necessary for the establishment of reversal is the measure of mobility. The extinction of the startle and orienting reflexes, conditional reflex formation, and conditional stimulus differentiation are the prerequisites of this procedure.

12. *Sleep inhibition:* Pavlov considered sleep to be a special form of inhibition and attributed a defensive, protective function to it. The experimental model he described is the twenty-seventh experiment in chapter 2, in which salivary secretion was conditioned to a faint sound. The unreinforced repetition of this weak conditional stimulus resulted in a decrease of salivary secretion and an inhibition that led to sleep. In human tests the same procedure is followed as in animal experiments. Voluntary, semivoluntary, and autonomic techniques are used. The number of stimulations required from the extinction of the conditional reflex to the occurrence of the first electroencephalographic signs of sleep is the indicator of this function. The extinction of the startle and orienting responses and conditional reflex formation and extinction are the prerequisites of this procedure.

By these twelve test procedures, experimentally approachable, first signal system functions in humans are revealed. In the next three test procedures (13, 14, 15) transmission from the first to the second signal system are exposed to examination.

TRANSMISSION FROM THE FIRST TO THE SECOND
SIGNAL SYSTEM

13. *Secondary conditional reflex to non-verbal conditional stimulus:* In this test a primary conditional reflex is conditioned to a secondary, non-verbal, conditional stimulus. Voluntary, semivoluntary, and autonomic techniques are used. The procedure here is similar to that described previously in test 10; after the conditional reflex to a conditional stimulus is well established, another stimulus is presented prior to the conditional stimulus. The number of associations required before the

conditional reflex develops to the second (non-verbal) conditional stimulus alone is the measure of this function.

14. *Conditional autonomic reflex to hetero-verbal conditional stimulus:* In this test an autonomic response is conditioned to a verbal command. The sensory–autonomic reflex is replaced by a verbal–autonomic reflex. As the first step of this test the unconditional sensory–autonomic pupillary (constriction) reflex to light is conditioned to an auditory (bell) stimulus. The primary conditional stimulus thereafter is combined with the squeezing by the subject of a dynamometer to the (heteroverbal) command "Contract." The number of associated administrations of stimuli (verbal command "Contract" and auditory bell) required before pupillary constriction develops to the verbal command is one of the measures of transmission from the first to the second signal system.

15. *Conditional motor reflex to heteroverbal conditional stimulus:* In this test a voluntary response is conditioned to a verbal stimulus. The sensory motor reflex is replaced by a verbal motor reflex. A modification of Ivanov-Smolensky's technique is used for this test. Pressing is conditioned to an auditory bell signal and reinforced with the word "Right." Thereafter, the bell signal is replaced by the corresponding verbal signal ("It rings"). The number of associated administrations of stimuli (bell and verbal) necessary before the motor reflex to the verbal conditional stimulus takes place is another measure of the transmission from the first to the second signal system.

Second signal system functioning is studied in the last three test procedures (16, 17, 18).

SECOND SIGNAL SYSTEM

16. *Transmission from heteroverbal to autoverbal conditional stimulus:* In this test an autonomic response to a heteroverbal stimulus is conditioned to an autoverbal stimulus. The verbal–autonomic reflex is replaced by an ideo-autonomic reflex. This procedure follows the same lines as described in test 14, in which the conditional autonomic reflex to the hetero-

verbal conditional stimulus was studied. In test 14 a light reflex was conditioned, at first to an auditory bell stimulus and thereafter to the heteroverbal command "Contract." As a further step in this test the command "Contract" is given by the subject himself, first loudly and then subvocally by thinking of it. The number of heteroverbal stimulus administrations required before the pupillary light reaction develops to the autoverbal stimulus is one of the measures of the transmission (from hetero- to autoverbal) in the second signal system.

17. *Transmission from heteroverbal stimulus to written symbol.* In this test a voluntary response to a verbal stimulus is conditioned to visual symbols. This test procedure is described among the conditioning techniques in which conditioning of voluntary activity in the study of second signal system processes is used. Here, a verbal signal, the word "Press," serves as the unconditional stimulus, and this voluntary activity is conditioned at first to the presentation of three lights of different colors in a specific order. Thereafter, the three lights, instead of being presented as visual stimuli, are verbalized (transmission from first to second signal system). When this is well established, the three lamps are neither flashed nor called verbally but their written symbols are projected. The number of heteroverbal stimuli required before squeezing of a balloon develops to the written symbol is another measure of the transmission (from heteroverbal to the visual symbol) in the second signal system.

18. *Word associations.* In this test a verbal response to a verbal stimulus is studied. Fifty to one hundred words seem to be sufficient for testing purposes. Reaction times are registered. Each individual response is fitted into the appropriate category. The evaluation of this test is shown on the next page.

The actual figure of each and the ratio between the different responses is the finest indicator of second signal system functioning.

On the basis of these diagnostic tests the concept of normal (psychological-physiological) is established in a statistical sense, and the abnormal deviation (pathological-psychopathological) can be qualitatively and quantitatively expressed.

Reaction Time
  Mean
  Median
Primitive Responses
  No Responses
    None (whatsoever)
    Startle response
    Autonomic responses
    Skeletomuscular movements or gestures
    Echolalic responses
    "Yes" responses
    Tautological responses
    Vague, meaningless responses
  Subtotal of no responses
  Negating Responses
    "No" responses
    Rejecting responses
  Subtotal of negating responses
  Extra-Signaling Responses
    Sound associations
    Incoherent reactions
    Neologisms
    Onomatopoeic responses
    Egocentric responses
    Delusional responses
  Subtotal of extra-signaling responses
  Subtotal of primitive responses
Transitional Responses
  Multiword responses
  "Yes" and adequate responses
  Repetition and adequate responses
  Subtotal of transitional responses
Higher Responses
  Individual concrete responses
  General concrete responses
  General abstract responses
  Subtotal of higher responses
  Total number of primitive and transitional responses
  Total number of transitional and higher responses
  Total number of responses

Since the different test procedures are connected with different neurophysiological functions, the behavioral tests reflect pathological processes in the brain.

PART FOUR

Conditioning in Psychiatry

9

GENERAL AND CLINICAL
PSYCHOPATHOLOGY

THE NEUROPHYSIOLOGICAL orientation in psychiatry opened new
leads in revealing the functional alterations in the background
of pathological behavior. Conditioning in psychiatry is linked
with both the behavioral and the neurophysiological approaches, the conditional reflex being a behavioral phenomenon
and a functioning pattern of the nervous system.

GENERAL PSYCHOPATHOLOGY

Classical psychiatry and, consequently, psychopathology
were based on detailed clinical descriptions. The conditioning
method, with the applicable human conditioning techniques
and procedures, extended the fields of observable phenomena
with experimental findings.

Personality development is differently conceived by the
different approaches. According to the classical school, at
birth only the autonomic centers are fully developed and
functioning in the central nervous system. Since the activity
of the exteroceptors of the early infant is insufficient, his internal, vital feelings are dominant. Exteroception develops pro-
gressively, and with it the collection of life experiences begins.
Sensorial perception leads to image formation, which consists
of picture-like reflections. With the full development of asso-
ciational paths, ideational processes begin, leading to abstract
thinking and the whole range of intellectual activity which
this allows.

Pavlov himself did not promote any theory of personality development. Nyirö, on Pavlovian grounds, believed that in the process of psychological development well-defined structural organizations are elaborated by the special interplay between the basic processes of excitation and inhibition and by the analytical and synthetical functioning of the central nervous system. These functional dynamic structures and the interaction between them are the basis of all psychological activity. Three structural organizations are described: cognitive, relational, and adaptive. In the development of all three structural organizations, differential inhibition plays a prominent role. Futhermore, functions of the cognitive structure influence relational functioning, and the interaction between these two also has an impetus on adaptive patterns. In turn, adaptation feeds back to cognitive and relational functions. The basis of these influences is induction, one of the fundamental patterns of central nervous system functioning.

The neurophysiological school correlates personality development with the physiological development of the central nervous system. Behavior is seen as "an expression of the functional capacity of the organism," which is the result of the functional capacities of the various central nervous system structures. Prenatal behavior was observed by Fitzgerald and Windle (1942) before Hooker conducted a systematic study and summarized his findings in a dissertation on the reflex activities of the human fetus (1943). Postnatal behavior was conceptualized by Gesell, who described the development of behavior in the different aspects of "growth," namely, in motor, adaptive, language, and personal social behavior. He believed that, ontogenetically, motor behavior is the oldest.

In the background of this functional progress there are structural developmental changes, as described by Bühler (1929). At birth the only paths ready are those which lead from the sense organs to the cortex, at first those for smell or taste, then for sight, and lastly those for hearing. The large motor paths that rise from the cortex and conduct impulses to the muscles are in an incipient developmental stage, and the multiple connecting paths are even less developed. The increase in size of the brain cells and the development of the conducting systems, together with the growth of connective tissue, result in a large weight increase of the cerebrum. Pfister has shown that in the first nine months of life the brain doubles in size and that it trebles before the end of the third year. Thus all the basic mental functions of the child are acquired in the first three or four years of life.

The concomitant psychological development is conceived differently by different authors. Bühler conceived it in three developmental levels: instinctual, training, and intellectual. Piaget distinguished among the sensomotor, the preoperative, the operative, and the formal phase of development. During this development the initially rigid, irreversible schemes of action and thought become pliable and reversible.

The experimental approach to psychiatry is based on neurophysiological findings but uses behavioral (verbal and nonverbal) measures.

Eysenck and his school attempted to establish the dimensions of personality and to develop the necessary psychological tests to measure those dimensions. At first, Eysenck, by a study using factor analysis, established what he thought to be the main factors of personality and thereafter searched for objective tests to measure those factors. In Eysenck's work, Jung's extroversion-introversion dichotomy, although used in a somewhat different sense, became quantifiable by tests in which the conditional reflex method was used. Eysenck presented two postulates. According to the first, human beings differ with respect to the speed with which excitation and inhibition are produced, the strength of the produced excitation and inhibition, and the speed with which inhibition is dissipated. According to the second postulate, individuals in whom excitation is generated slowly and in whom the excitation is relatively weak develop extroverted patterns of behavior, while those in whom excitation is generated quickly and in whom the excitation is strong develop introverted patterns of behavior. Similarly, those in whom inhibition is generated quickly and in whom this inhibition is strong and can be slowly dissipated are predisposed to introverted behavioral patterns. On these theoretical grounds Eysenck states that introverts form conditional reflexes quickly and extinguish them slowly, while extroverts form conditional reflexes slowly but extinguish them quickly. Frank's study with the eyelid closure technique supported Eysenck's findings.

Another approach in defining personality in experimental terms is based on the assumption that personality is a synthetic concept, embracing all the psychological and somatic properties of the human organism, the whole active individual from birth to death. Thus, personality is expressed by the sum of the possible unconditional reflexes and first and second signaling system conditional reflexes. The whole of central nervous system functioning is understood by "personality."

Pavlov understood consciousness as the nervous activity of a certain part of the cerebral hemispheres, which possesses, at a given moment, optimal excitability with maximal excitatory state, while the excitability and the excitatory state of the other peripheral parts of the cerebral hemisphere are diminished. At this point, new conditional reflexes are easily formed and differentiation develops successfully.

Memory, another complex psychological function, was studied intensively and correlated with findings on conditional reflex tests (Gantt, Solyom, etc.). In general, a direct relationship was found between memory function and conditioning ability, which means that subjects with a good memory in general are conditioned faster. The different aspects of memory can be tested, that is, acquisition by new conditional reflex formation, retention by trace and delayed reflex formation, and recall by second signal system tests.

Attention is correlated with the arousal functioning of the brain stem reticular formation. It is tested by the persistence of the orienting reflex. This persistence is directly proportionate to the level of vigilance, and inversely with tenacity. In other words, the higher the level of vigilance, the more difficult it becomes to extinguish the orienting reflex and, the lower the level of vigilance, the more difficult it becomes to obtain a startle response.

The different levels of the cognitive structural organization can also be measured by test procedures.

Diffuse sensation can be tested by the orienting response test: differentiated perception by conditional reflex formation and conditional stimulus differentiation. Ideational processes can be tested by word association tests.

In the affective area, quantification of anxiety was of major interest for some time. Physiological and pathological anxiety were discriminated. Welch and Kubis repeatedly found that up to a certain point the degree of anxiety is positively related to the rate of conditioning ability; the higher the anxiety level, the fewer the trials necessary for the establishment of the conditional reflex. The extinction of the orienting reflex becomes increasingly difficult on higher anxiety levels. Spence and Bancroft believe that differentiation is also positively related to a limited degree of fear, which means that differentiation takes place significantly sooner in fear-producing situations. In the case of pathological anxiety, it was found that subjects show less discrimination. The extinction rate of the orienting reflex in subjects with dysthymic mood change (depression) is low. Similarly, conditioning ability, discrimination, and other first signal system activities function at a low level. The transmission from the first to the second signal system is slow, and word association time is prolonged. With increasing severity of the clinical condition, the quality of word associations is first altered, then the function of differentiation becomes impaired, before conditioning ability is interfered with. In the acute manic syndrome, the orienting reflex becomes unextinguishable.

The extinction of the orienting reflex is of primary importance in the pathology of adaptive functioning. Conditioning ability of the different autonomic functions, of voluntary activity, and of semivoluntary automatisms, together with the conditioning of verbal behavior, supply essential information on this functioning. Unconditional and conditional reflexes and verbal responses describe adaptive behavior adequately. In the case of hyperthymic mood, the extinction of the orienting reflex becomes increasingly difficult but conditional reflexes are formed with ease and differentiation is prompt. The transmission from the first to the second signal system is fast and word association time short.

Psychological functioning thus became approachable by psychophysiological tests, in which behavioral manifestations with a well-defined neurophysiological—pathological—basis are measured. General psychopathology progressed from a descriptive to an experimental stage, in which direct descriptive observation was supplemented by instrumentally quantified registration.

CLINICAL PSYCHOPATHOLOGY

The conditional reflex method and the various techniques applicable in diagnostic test procedures widened the scope of information on the different clinical psychiatric conditions. What follows is a description of some of the clinical syndromes on the basis of their conditional reflex patterns.

Mental Deficiency

Mental deficiency is defined as a condition of arrested or incomplete development of mind existing before the age of eighteen years, irrespective of cause (Gregory 1961). A mental defective is a person lacking intelligence to the degree that he cannot make an average adjustment to life. Depending on the degree of retardation, mental defectives are grouped into three categories: morons, imbeciles, and idiots.

The three groups differ from one another in their degree of social adaptation. No social adaptation is found in the idiot group, passive adaptation in the imbecilic, and a limited active adaptation in morons. This indicates that, while the idiot does not participate in social activities, imbeciles do in a passive manner and morons do actively but on a limited basis.

The three groups can be differentiated by psychological means. On the basis of I.Q. tests (Binet-Simon, Wechsler-Bellevue), mental defectives with an I.Q. of 20 or lower are considered idiots, those from 20–49 imbeciles, and those from 50–69 morons.

Conditioning test procedures revealed the following findings:

a) *Unconditional reflex behavior:* Unconditional reflex activity is normal in most of the groups of mental defectives. However, Astrup found occasionally a partial inhibition of the motor and autonomic reactions to electrical current. On this basis, and on Popper's findings that some mental defectives show great endurance to pain, it was surmised that unconditional reflex activity is impaired in some of these patients.

b) *Orienting reflex behavior:* No orienting reflex, or an extremely weak persistence of the orienting reflex was found, indicating a low arousal level, which confirms Hernandez-Peon's neurophysiological hypothesis that a low arousal level, and, consequently attention level, form the basis of mental deficiency.

c) *Conditional reflex behavior:* Conditional reflex formation takes a tedious, long course. Significantly, greater numbers of combined presentations of conditional stimuli and unconditional stimuli are required than in normals to establish the conditional reflex. Conditional stimulus generalization and differentiation are impaired. Secondary conditional reflexes cannot be formed in idiots at all and only with great difficulty in imbeciles and morons.

d) *Transmission from first to second signal system:* In the two higher grades of defectives transmission from the first to the second signal system succeeds slowly.

e) *Verbal behavior:* Characteristic word associates are found. Nathan described a prolongation in time; Sommer, a poverty of responses; and Astrup revealed that imbeciles give mainly primitive and morons mainly transitional responses.

Organic Brain Syndromes

"Organic brain syndrome" refers to that constellation of psychiatric symptoms which is associated with morphological, macroscopic, or microscopic alterations in the central nervous system. These symptoms are generally defined as clouding of consciousness, dysmnesia, and dementia (Mayer-Gross, Slater, and Roth).

The establishment of the diagnosis of organic brain syndrome (acute or chronic) follows different lines. By social criteria, the acute brain syndrome is characterized by reversibility of decompensation in social adaptation, and the chronic brain syndrome is seen as a progressive decline in social performance. Psychologically, the diagnosis is made through test procedures (i.e. Bender–Gestalt, etc.). Psychiatric criteria are the prominence of a clouded state of consciousness in acute cases and the prominence of progressive dementia in chronic cases.

Since behavioral conditional reflex test procedures reveal neurophysiological alterations, they are also applicable for detecting organicity (Astrup, Balonov, Chistovich, Traugott). The following findings were described in the different conditions:

1. *Acute brain syndrome:* All first and second signal system activity functions at a lower level.
2. *Aging:* It was indicated that there is a difference in the acquisition and the extinction of conditional reflexes between the various age groups (Botwinick, Kornetsky, Brown, Geiselhart, etc.); Solyom found a persistence of the orienting reflex, decreased conditioning ability, and differentiation in normal old subjects.
3. *Chronic brain syndrome:*
    a) *Senile dementia:* There is generally decreased activity, manifested in decreased conditioning ability and increased extinction rate of the conditional reflex (Cameron, etc.).
    b) *Presenile dementias (Alzheimer's and Pick's diseases):* Conditioning ability is significantly decreased (Gantt, Muncie, etc.).
    c) *Korsakoff's syndrome:* Conditional reflex formation (and retention) and conditional stimulus differentiation are impaired (Gantt, Linsky, Solyom, etc.).

The impairment of conditional reflex activity in the case of an acute brain syndrome is reversible and decreases with time. The opposite applies to a chronic brain syndrome, in which the impairment is irreversible and increases as time passes.

Paranoid Psychoses

Paranoia is defined as a disorder characterized by fixed systematized delusions, with the absence of hallucinations and the preservation of logical thinking. The word "paranoid" has been used for conditions resembling paranoia (Valentine 1962).

Paranoia can be diagnosed on social, psychological, or psychiatric grounds. The inadequate social behavior of the paranoid in certain situations appears to be in great contrast to his otherwise intact personality patterns. Thus, the delusional psychotic material may remain long hidden.

On the basis of conditional reflex studies, Astrup divided paranoid schizophrenic patients into two categories. In the first group he placed those paranoid cases who were dominated by projection symptoms. The characteristic findings in these patients were as follows:

a) *Unconditional reflex behavior:* After instruction, more than one-quarter of the cases failed to withdraw the finger tip to avoid electroshock in one or more trials, and in about half of the cases a tendency to inhibit the unconditional reflex was revealed. The latter finding reached high statistical significance when compared to other functional psychoses.

b) *Conditional reflex behavior:* Conditioning ability was not essentially different from normals, but extinction and differentiation of conditional stimuli were impaired in approximately 25 per cent of the patients. The same percentage failed to reverse the negative reflex into a positive, whereas somewhat fewer patients failed to reverse the positive reflex into a negative.

c) *Verbal behavior:* Increased association time was found in more than 40 per cent of the cases, and in a high percentage echolalic and multiword responses were obtained.

In the second group of paranoid schizophrenics, Astrup enrolled patients with systematized delusions. The conditional reflex profile of these patients as compared to the first paranoid group is as follows:

a) *Unconditional reflex behavior:* The tendency to inhibit the unconditional reflex is weaker.

b) *Conditional reflex behavior:* Similar to the first group.

c) *Verbal behavior:* Increased association time was found in more than 50 per cent of the patients, and even a higher percentage gave echolalic and multiword responses. More intensive second signal system pathology was found in this group of paranoid patients.

In summary: Diagnostic test procedures in paranoid psychoses revealed occasionally weak unconditional reflexes, impaired internal inhibitory functions (extinction, differentiation), prolonged word association time with a relatively high number of transitional responses.

Manic-Depressive Psychosis

The diagnosis of manic-depressive psychosis is established on the basis of the three characteristics of the illness: the primary disturbance of mood, the persistent recurrence of the moods, and complete recovery between attacks.

Several authors contributed to the conditional reflex profile of this illness (Faddeyeva, Ivanov-Smolensky, Protopopov, etc.). On the basis of their work the following findings were registered.

a) *Unconditional reflex behavior:* Reaction time is short in manic conditions, prolonged in depressions, and reactions are strong and weak, respectively.

b) *Orienting reflex behavior:* The orienting reflex is persistent in manic conditions and non-persistent in depressions.

c) *Conditional reflex behavior:* Conditioning ability increases (or beyond a certain level becomes impossible) in manic conditions and decreases in depressions; delayed and trace reflexes are impaired in both.

d) *Transmission from first to second signal system:* This transmission increases (or beyond a certain level becomes impossible) in manic conditions and decreases in depressions.

e) *Verbal behavior:* Word association time is decreased in manic conditions (Moravcsik, Ivanov-Smolensky) and increases in depressions (Birnbaum). The number of responses decreases in depressions; echolalic, tautological, vague, meaningless responses and sound associations are increased in manics (Aschaffenburg, Soserlin, Kilian). Manic patients give also a greater number of transitional—multiword—responses (Astrup).

Schizophrenia

Bleuler conceived schizophrenia as a group of disease processes. Further classifications were Langfeldt's, which subdivided schizophrenias into processual and reactive types, and Leonhard's, which was similar to Kleist's but without full acceptance of the latter's localization theory and remaining on the level of clinical description.

A neurophysiological theory of schizophrenia in the frame of reference of conditioning theory was presented by Bridger. This was based on the assumption that the common feature in sleep, hypnosis, sensory isolation, sleep deprivation, and so on, is neocortical inhibition and limbic lobe excitation. He indicated that the neocortex is the morphological substrate that discriminates the conditional stimulus from the unconditional stimulus. The limbic lobe has not developed this function of discrimination of stimuli. Thus neocortical inhibition and limbic system excitation may produce a confusion between the symbol and the object symbolized. This disturbance manifests itself in hallucinations, delusions, and other symptoms found in schizophrenics.

A systematic conditional reflex study in schizophrenia was carried out by Astrup (1962). Prior to this the following were the most revealing findings.

a) *Unconditional reflex behavior:* Ivanov-Smolensky found the unconditional defensive reflex occasionally inhibited in some of the catatonic patients.

b) *Orienting reflex behavior:* Occasionally no orienting reflex was obtained in the same group of patients (Ivanov-Smolensky).

c) *Conditional reflex behavior:* Dobrzhanskaya found marked changes in conditional reflex functioning from time to time in acute schizophrenics. Several workers indicated impaired conditioning ability and conditional stimulus differentiation (Gantt, Vinogradov and Raiser, Peters and Murphree, etc.). Ivanov-Smolensky claimed that the ability to form conditional reflexes is very different in the various areas. For example, he found it impossible to form motor conditional reflexes, while he was able to establish conditional respiratory or vascular responses. Others revealed a generally impaired internal inhibition (Chuchmareva, Rushkevich, Sinkevich, etc.). Kutsin was able to subdivide chronic schizophrenic patients into two groups. In one group he found a marked weakness of both excitatory and inhibitory processes; in the other, only slight conditional reflex changes compared to normal.

d) *Interaction between the two signal systems:* Several authors found disassociation in the interaction of the first and second signal system in general (Vinogradov, Reiter, Kaufner, etc.). Others found this primarily in the paranoids.

Astrup used Langfeldt's and Schneider's principles in the classification of the acute cases and Leonhard's in the chronic cases in his study. Thus, he grouped (*a*) acute and subacute schizophrenics as hebephrenic and hebephrenic-paranoid cases, (*b*) catatonic and mixed catatonic cases, (*c*) paranoid cases with projection symptoms, and (*d*) paranoid cases with systematized delusions.

Astrup tested each of these categories and subgroups with a standardized test procedure that supplied information on first and second signal system activity and also on the interaction of the two systems. In his test procedure he used the finger-withdrawal technique, plethysmography, the conditional motor reflex with verbal reinforcement, and the word association test with fifty words. He found distinct differences between the different categories and groups and, on the basis of his study, considered the following six factors to be important neurophysiological mechanisms in schizophrenics: inhibition of subcortical centers; induced disinhibitions and excitations; dissociations related to subcortical inhibition; impairment of internal inhibition; inertia of nervous processes; weakness of internal inhibition as the evolutionally latest developed and most vulnerable process. Astrup's study also revealed that the inhibitory tendency of unconditional reflexes and the presence of dissociative phenomena parallel the schizophrenic's deterioration.

Gantt has pointed out that there may be a split in the interactions of nervous functions in schizophrenics. This dissociation he called "schizokinesis." He considered it as an inherent conflict between the general basic emotional response and the more adaptive responses. On the other hand, he considered "autokinesis" to be the ability of the organism to form new patterns of behavior without external stimulation. There was also some indication in Astrup's study that the disturbances of the higher nervous activity in schizophrenia might be explained on the basis of the neurophysiological principles of autokinesis and schizokinesis—in other words, that the disturbance develops along certain pathways relatively independent of the precipitating factors and determined by heredity.

In general, the following changes are to be found in schizophrenics in conditional reflex test procedures:

a) *Unconditional reflex behavior:* Unconditional reflexes are increasingly inhibited as the schizophrenic process progresses. In some patients with catatonic stupor some of the unconditional reflexes are absent.

b) *Orienting reflex behavior:* There is an increased persistence of the orienting reflex in most of the acute cases and decreased persistence in the chronic deteriorated cases. In some catatonic patients the orienting reflex is absent.

c) *Conditional reflex behavior:* With the progress of the illness, conditioning ability decreases; similarly, internal inhibitory functions (extinction, differentiation, delayed and trace reflex formation). Sleep inhibition develops to repetitive administration of the same conditional stimulus in most schizophrenics faster than it does in normals.

d) *Interaction between the two signal systems:* The transmission function from the first to the second signal system is impaired. Owing to this impairment and to dissociative phenomena, the second signal system functions independently from the first, as manifested in intensive and varied second signal system pathology with relatively intact first signal system functioning.

e) *Verbal behavior:* Changes in word association tests parallel severity of the illness. Association time, which is markedly prolonged in serious conditions, is a fine indicator of the clinical changes. In catatonic conditions the number of verbal responses decreases. In hebephrenics there is in general a decrease of higher responses and an increase of primitive responses, among them the "Yes," vague, meaningless, incoherent, sound association responses. In paranoid cases the reply "No" or rejecting responses are more frequent, together with egocentric and delusional responses. In simple schizophrenics "Yes" replies and tautological and multiword responses are increased. While in the acute form of the illness there is a considerable number of higher reactions, and neologisms occur just occasionally, in chronic cases there is a progressive change from the general abstract to the general concrete, then to the individual concrete, and finally to cessation of higher responses and an increase in neologisms and onomatopoeic responses.

Neurosis

The difference between neurosis and psychosis has been the subject of great controversy in the literature. Some believe that a difference exists between the two, others prefer to see both as part of a continuum.

Conditional reflex studies in neurotics have not revealed any homogeneous findings. The first impression that neurotics condition less readily than do normals (Peters and Murphy, Kubis) was not confirmed by further studies. Neither could other studies, which indicated that neurotics condition more readily than do normals and psychotics more readily than neurotics (Spence and Taylor, Howe), be supported. Astrup found that the general disturbance in neurotics is often small and within the range of normal variation. On the other hand, there is a marked deviation from the normal when the different neurotic conditions are individually investigated.

a) *Neurasthenia* is subdivided by Ivanov-Smolensky into three consecutive stages. In the first stage great irritability and lack of capacity to inhibit actions and emotions are characteristic. Using conditional reflex tests, he found a weakness of the internal inhibitory functions. In the second stage he found a lability of the excitatory process, manifested in easily changeable conditional reflex functions. Thereafter, with the increasing incapacity to work, the weakness of the excitatory process and the predominance of the inhibitory processes develop. In chronic conditions, a tendency to sleep inhibition prevails.

b) In *hysteria*, according to Faddeyeva and Povorinsky, the main alteration is manifested in the tendency to develop sleep inhibition promptly. Seredina and Rajeva discovered an impairment in the transmission function from the first to the second signal system. Others found that in hysterical fits the conditional reflexes are inhibited similarly to the epileptic *grand mal* seizures, but conditioning ability remains intact in hysterics during the convulsions, and the developed conditional reflex can be elicited in the postconvulsion state. In hysterical blindness the conditional reflex to visual conditional stimulus alone is inhibited, but, if the visual signal precedes an auditory conditional stimulus, the latency period of the conditional reflex to the auditory signal is shortened, showing that the visual signal has a function in conditioning procedure. Such is not the case in organic blindness. Astrup found the verbal reactions in some of the hysterics severely inhibited.

c) In *phobias* Seredina found a weakness of the internal inhibitory processes; Belousova found a tendency to sleep inhibition.

Conditional reflex test procedures revealed the following changes in the neuroses.

a) *Unconditional reflex behavior:* Autonomic reactivity in general tends to be increased, hence the decrease in skin resistance to an electroshock, etc. On the other hand, in some hysterics, those with functional anesthesia, no unconditional reflex can be elicited from the specific area.

b) *Orienting reflex behavior:* The persistence of the orienting reflex is increased in anxiety and decreased in neurotic depressive reaction.

c) *Conditional reflex behavior:* Conditioning ability is increased in general. On the other hand, delayed and trace reflexes are impaired. In phobic reactions there is a specifically increased tendency of generalization with the lack of differentiation.

d) *Verbal behavior:* In word association tests, neurotics react like normals. Occasionally, there is an increase in multiword responses in anxiety or an increase in reaction time in depressive reactions.

Changes revealed by conditional reflex test procedures in the different clinical conditions are generally described in Astrup's book *Conditional Reflex Studies in Schizophrenia.*

10

TREATMENT IN

PSYCHIATRY

IT IS COMMON TO distinguish between causal and symptomatic therapies. A therapy is considered causal if the known etiology of an illness is being treated and symptomatic if its manifestations are the objects of the treatment process. Since the etiologies of the most important psychiatric illnesses have remained basically unknown, the symptomatic therapies are the best available in present-day psychiatry. These are psychotherapy, behavior therapy, and the physical therapies (including pharmacotherapy).

PSYCHOTHERAPY

Psychotherapy refers to the method of treating the mentally ill by psychological means (Unger) or without physical means (Lehmann).

Conditioning theory supplies a basis for psychotherapeutic procedures. According to Pavlov, "the word is as real a conditional stimulus as all the other stimuli we have in common with animals, but at the same time more all-embracing than any of the other stimuli."

Platonov's psychotherapeutic method is based on the assumption that, on the one hand, the word may replace, reflect, or generalize the meaning of the concrete stimuli of the external or internal environment, while, on the other hand, a complex system of abstract ideas has been created based entirely on "word signalization," a system that has continuity through the history of man. The verbal stimulus can lead to simple and complex physiological reactions, and, depending on the meaning with which the word is charged, it may evoke a positive, negative, or even perverted reactive development. Platonov's experiments suggested the possibility of influencing different physical functions, even immunological processes of the organism, by words.

Platonov interpreted the physiological mechanisms underlying psychotherapy on classical Pavlovian lines. He considered the cerebral cortex as the organ that receives all the stimuli from the external (exteroceptive) and internal (interoceptive) worlds and that establishes the bonds between these stimuli. This makes clear why the nature of the functioning of the internal organs and systems depends on the tone of the cerebral cortex, on the state of equilibrium of the basic cortical processes, and on the proper functional relationship between the cerebral cortex and the subcortical area. It also explains why the treatment of the functional state of the cerebral cortex leads to normalization of the activity of the affected internal organs or systems.

On Pavlovian grounds, Platonov considered emotion as a subcortical function and thought that the adequate "tone" of the cortex is maintained by the emotion supplied from the adjacent subcortex. On the other hand, the active state of the cerebral cortex negatively inducts the subcortex and inhibits its activity, while the inhibited state of the cortex positively inducts the subcortex and increases its general activity.

In psychotherapy, thus, by using "suggested emotions," the tone of the cerebral cortex is altered. This in turn exerts a control over the entire organism.

According to Platonov, psychobiologically based psychotherapy represents active interference on the part of the physician, who can alter the state of the patient's corticosubcortical dynamics. Therefore he claims that psychotherapy should first reveal the specific conditions predisposing and provoking the neurosis. The aim of psychotherapy is to remove the factors that have functionally weakened the cerebral cortex and to contribute to raising the general tone of the cortex. The different psychotherapeutic means for this purpose are (*a*) the affirmative (imperative) suggestion in waking or in hypnotic state, (*b*) the influence by word on the conscious level (persuasion, explanation) or during suggested drowsiness or sleep, and (*c*) the extensive anamnestic analysis of the patient's higher nervous activity. In the combined method applied by Platonov, therapy begins with a series of anamnestic interviews that establishes a positive contact between physician and patient, followed by explanation and persuasion (psychotherapy on the conscious level), then by suggestion under hypnosis to consolidate what has been said on the conscious level. The final stage in this combined method is suggested rest in the same hypnotic state that was used for suggestion.

By Platonov's method words became "a physiological and therapeutic" factor. The recognition that the word is a conditional stimulus and "owing to the entire proceeding life of the human adult a word is connected with all the external and internal stimuli coming to the cerebral hemispheres, signals all of them, replaces all of them and can therefore, evoke all the actions and reactions of the organism which these stimuli produce" (Pavlov) is one of the most valid and practically useful contributions that has been made to medical therapy "without physical means."

BEHAVIOR THERAPY

In the classical experiments of Pavlov, conditional reflex formation was described as the associated administration of the conditional and unconditional stimuli, in that order. The conditional reflex is a specific type of learning in this case, but learning does not necessarily follow the patterns of classical conditioning. In other words, while something new is acquired during every learning procedure, as during the conditioning procedure, in some of the learnings this acquisition is not the result of the association of a conditional and an unconditional stimulus. In 1928 Miller and Konorski described a type of conditioning in which the establishment of the conditional reflex was not entirely dependent on the repeated association of the two stimuli, but was also dependent on a third motivational factor. In this instrumental conditioning the subject receives the reward or avoids the punishment only if he makes the correct, that is, the conditioned, response.

Modern learning theories (contiguity and reinforcement theories) utilize both the classical and the instrumental conditioning models. Contiguity theory as represented by Tolman and Guthrie uses the classical model and holds the view that the basic condition necessary for learning is that of contiguity of experience.

Tolman conceived of learning as the acquisition of information about the environment and considered contiguity, the spatial and temporal patterning of stimulus events, as the necessary requisite. Similarly, Guthrie thought that simultaneity of stimulus cues and responses is all that is required for acquisition. Reinforcement theory uses the instrumental conditioning model. According to Hull, if in the course of trial and error responses the organism performs the response that is associated with the reduction of motivation, the probability that this response will occur again under similar conditions increases. He considered the concept of drive reduction crucial and designated it as the law of effect or the principle of reinforcement.

On the basis of a long series of studies Schlosberg concluded (1937) that there are two types of learning. One of these has to do with autonomically mediated visceral reactions, which follow the principle of association or sheer contiguity based on classical conditioning. The other type of learning, according to Schlosberg, has to do with more "precise adaptive responses" of the skeletal muscles. This learning follows the principle of success or reinforcement based on the principles of instrumental conditioning. Schlosberg's two-factor theory was further elaborated by Skinner, who distinguished between preparatory (Type S) and consummatory (Type R) conditioning. In Type S the unconditional stimulus is correlated with the conditional stimulus, whereas in Type R the unconditional stimulus is correlated with the response. On the basis of experiments,

Skinner concludes that while autonomically mediated (i.e., emotional) reactions are learned on the basis of contiguity utilizing Type S conditioning, mediated skeletal muscle responses are learned on the basis of reinforcement utilizing Type R conditioning.

Behavior therapy was developed on the basis of modern learning theory, not conditioning theory. Application of the principles of learning theory suggested that neurotic symptoms in general are learned unadaptive patterns of behavior. Or, more precisely, the different neurotic symptoms labeled as different neurotic disorders are unadaptive behavior conditioned to certain classes of stimuli. Thus behavior therapy concentrates on the extinction of these unadaptive conditioned responses.

Eysenck summarized the ten most important characteristics of behavior therapy. According to him, behavior therapy is based on consistent, properly formulated theory leading to stable deductions (1). It is derived from experimental studies specifically designated to test basic theory and deductions made therefrom (2). Behavior therapy is based on the hypothesis that symptoms are unadaptive conditional responses (3) and are regarded as faulty learning (4). Furthermore, it believes that symptomatology is determined by individual differences in conditionability and autonomic lability, as well as accidental environmental circumstances (5). Behavior therapy considers the historical development of neurotic disorders, from the point of view of treatment, irrelevant and is concerned with habits existing at the actual present (6). Therapy deals with the treatment of the symptom itself by extinguishing unadaptive conditional reflexes and establishing desirable conditional reflexes (7). This symptomatic treatment leads to permanent recovery (8) without interpretations (9) and personal relations (10) utilized in the therapeutic situation.

The four practiced behavior therapeutic techniques are (a) therapy by positive conditioning, (b) reciprocal inhibition therapy, (c) therapy by negative practice, and (d) aversion therapy.

a) Therapy by positive conditioning is indicated in cases

in whom there are deficient conditioned reactions or, more precisely, in cases with the absence of some or one specific good (adaptive) habit. Bed-wetting is the prototype of this condition. This therapy has been successfully applied in cases of enuresis. At the beginning of micturation the ringing of the bell awakes the sleeping subject. Awakening, as an external inhibition, stops micturation. Thus, by repetition, micturation is postponed and the maladaptive conditional reflex (habit) is replaced by a desirable conditional reflex (habit). This technique was first developed by Mowrer (1938) and extensively applied by Jones. Therapy by positive conditioning is also indicated in hysterical anesthesia, analgesia, and astereognosis (Sears and Cohen 1933) and was successfully applied by Malmo, Davis, and Barza in the case of a total hysterical deafness (1952). In these conditions an unconditional stimulus administered to an uninvolved sensory receptor is preceded by a conditional stimulus administered through the involved receptor. After a considerable number of associations the unadaptive conditional reflex (habit) is replaced by the desired conditional reflex.

b) Reciprocal inhibition therapy was developed by Wolpe (1947–48). While therapy by positive conditioning is indicated when there are deficient conditioned reactions, therapy by reciprocal inhibition is indicated in neurotic conditions characterized by "surplus" conditional reflexes, as, for example, in the anxiety reactions.

Wolpe described anxiety as the autonomic response patterns that are characteristically part of the given organism's response to noxious stimulation. He considered an anxiety response neurotic (unadaptive) when evoked in circumstances in which there is objectively no threat.

Reciprocal inhibition therapy as introduced by Wolpe is based on Sherrington's concept of reciprocal inhibition. According to this concept, with the activity of the agonist muscles there is a simultaneous inhibition of the antagonists. On the same basis Wolpe suggested that if a response incompatible with anxiety can be made to occur in the presence of anxiety-evoking stimuli, it will weaken the bond between these stimuli and the anxiety responses. Wolpe's animal experiments confirmed his expectations, and he found, for example, an antagonism between the anxiety responses and the feeding responses. In these experiments, as long as anxiety was strong enough to inhibit feeding, anxiety continued to be dominant, but when conditions were so changed that the feeding tendency became relatively stronger, the tendency to respond by anxiety to stimuli was gradually weakened.

Thus Wolpe applied eight different responses incompatible with anxiety in the presence of anxiety-evoking stimuli. These responses were assertive responses, sexual responses, relaxation responses, conditioned avoidance responses, feeding responses, respiratory responses, interview-induced emotional responses, and abreactions.

c) The principle of negative practice was developed by Dunlap (1932). He formulated the possible role of repetition in habit formation in three hypotheses. According to the alpha hypothesis, a response to a given stimulus increases the probability of the recurrence of the same response to the same, or substantially the same, stimulus. However, while practicing previously learned "wrong" responses, he found that the same "wrong" response at a certain point, instead of recurring, dropped out. The beta and gamma hypotheses he added on the basis of this observation. According to the beta hypothesis, repetition has no effect on the probable recurrence of a response except insofar as other factors operate through it. Furthermore, in the gamma hypothesis Dunlap stated that repetition does not increase, but, on the contrary, decreases, the probability of the recurrence of the response with the repetition of the same stimulus pattern.

It is the beta hypothesis on which the technique of negative practice is based. In other words, the motivation may operate through repetition toward the goal of maintaining a response or habit, or it may operate through repetition toward the elimination of a response or habit. The negative motivation— the desire of the patient to cure the habit—is utilized in negative practice for decreasing the probability of recurrence of the response, for the abolition of habit.

Negative practice is used in the treatment of habitual errors and is primarily indicated in so-called "habit residuals." Thus negative practice is successfully employed in stuttering and tics and also in correcting typing and piano errors. Beneficial effect was also claimed by Dunlap in speech block, enuresis, homosexuality, and masturbation. In the actual therapeutic application the patient is informed about the procedure and his co-operation is asked. Thereafter, conversation is carried out but interrupted as the behavioral symptom (stuttering, tics, etc.) appears. Then the patient is asked to repeat the mistake he has made.

The rationale of negative practice is not firmly established. Pavlov (1926) said that under certain circumstances conditional reflexes lose their strength in spite of being reinforced. He interpreted this by implying that conditional stimuli, after a considerable number of repetitions, produce a state of inhibition. In practice, when conditional stimuli are applied at short intervals, this inhibition develops faster. Similarly to Pavlov, Gardner and Nissen found (1948) that repetition of habits can lead to worsening or fading of performance, and Razran also noticed (1956) that "over-reinforcement" operates as a markedly negative factor. In explaining negative practice, Kendrick (1958) applied the term "inhibition with reinforcement," in which extinction of the habit is brought about by a habit of not responding, meaning that what is repeated in negative practice is just the motor aspect of the actual response involved in the habit or, in other words, the behavioral patterns of the habitual response without the affective and ideational components involved in the habit. The mechanism involved in the action, namely, that the new response extinguished the faulty learned behavioral pattern, Kendrick compared to the mechanism of conditional inhibition.

In all the therapies by negative practice, faulty (neither deficient nor surplus conditional reactions) behavioral responses are treated on the basis of a not fully understood mechanism.

d) Among the different behavioral techniques aversion therapy has been the most widely used. It is indicated and used in the treatment of alcoholism (Ichok 1934, Galant

1936), among the sexual aberrations in fetishism (Raymond 1956), homosexuality (Freund 1938), writer's cramp (Liversedge and Sylvester 1955), and several other conditions.

In the treatment of alcoholism the usual way of producing a conditioned aversion is by the administration of some nausea-inducing drug (apomorphine, emetin) prior to alcohol administration. Increasing evidence suggests that conditioned aversion can be produced, aside from the nausea-producing apomorphine, by all sorts of other stimuli, as, for example, by electroshock. In alcoholism, the alcohol administration is associated with apomorphine-produced nausea or with electroshock; in fetishism, the fetishistic object; in homosexuals, the projection of slides of undressed subjects of the same sex are given a negative valence in a similar manner. In writer's cramp, a special training apparatus was constructed to administer an electroshock in the case of tremor or spasm, which is in the center of this motor disorder.

Aversion therapy follows the principles of Hull's reinforcement theory in learning and as such is based on Konorski's instrumental conditioning model, in which a negative motivation, punishment, is applied for the extinction (negative reinforcement) of the unadaptive habit. In accordance with the two-factor theory, motor habits develop by reinforcement through instrumental conditioning, while autonomic habit by contiguity develops through classical conditioning. Thus, by aversion therapy, which utilizes the instrumental conditioning model, the primary symptom, the motor habit, is treated. The concomitant autonomic habit is to be dealt with simultaneously (reciprocal inhibition, etc., therapy).

These are the four most widely used behavioral therapeutic means, successful in the different clinical conditions in which the basic alteration is on the level of overt behavior and neurophysiology.

The primary indications for the different techniques established so far are as follows: positive conditioning: enuresis and conversion reactions; reciprocal inhibition: anxiety reactions and phobic reactions; negative practice: stuttering and tics; aversion therapy: alcoholism, sexual aberrations.

PHYSICAL THERAPIES

In the behavior therapies the mechanism involved in treatment counteracts manifestations developing primarily from the behavioral to the neurophysiological level of organization. On the other hand, in the physical therapies the mechanism involved in the treatment counteracts primarily neurophysiological manifestations, or those developing from the neurophysiological to the neurochemical level of organization.

The physical therapies are convulsive therapy, insulin coma, leucotomy, and drug therapy. Convulsive therapy is conducted by several means (electroshock, etc.).

In conditional reflex studies it was found that convulsive therapy leads to the temporary predominance of the activity of the lower central nervous system centers (Rosen and Gantt). In a systematic study on the effect of electroconvulsive therapy on reflex activity, it was found that during the period of convulsion, and for a limited time afterward, there is for a short time a temporary inhibition of unconditional reflexes and of the conditional reflexes. This period was found to extend to approximately twenty minutes (Lunn). The restoration of reflex activity was studied by Traugott, who found that the unconditional reflex is the first to be restored, followed by the first signal system conditional reflex activity, and immediately thereafter the second signal system activity. During the restoration of reactions in the second signal system he observed the following order: (a) verbal stimulus, autonomic or skeletomuscular response; (b) nonverbal stimulus, verbal response; and (c) verbal stimulus, verbal response. Association time is prolonged but gradually decreases, and, similarly, the increased proportion of primitive associations diminishes. In the follow-up conditional reflex studies on patients who had undergone electroconvulsive treatment, the normalization of the pattern on the different conditional reflex tests corresponded with the clinical improvement.

Insulin coma is induced by the parenteral administration of

insulin. While electroconvulsive therapy produced a temporary general weakening of the excitatory process (decrease of excitatory conditional reflexes) and weakening of the active cortical inhibition (loss of inhibitory reflexes, lack of differentiation, lengthening of the latency period), insulin coma therapy showed its effects only on the inhibitory conditional reflexes and not on the excitatory conditional reflexes (Gellhorn). However, during the period of coma there is a decreased unconditional reflex and an inhibited conditional reflex activity. The restoration period follows the same course as in electroconvulsive therapy, and in the follow-up the normalization of the patterns on the different conditional reflex tests also corresponds with the clinical improvement.

Leucotomy as a surgical procedure is today even more rarely applied than insulin coma therapy. It leads to a pronounced inertia of both the basic processes, that is, excitation and inhibition (Astrup).

The presently most widely employed physical therapies are the pharmacotherapies. Drug action is conceptualized in models using chemical, physiological, behavioral, and clinical frames of reference.

In the chemical model, drug action is described on the molecular level. Emphasis is placed on the interaction of psychotropic drugs with tryptophan and phenylalanin metabolism, with acetylcholine formation and destruction, etc. (Brodie, Heath, Hoagland, Hoffer, Marazzi, Prochop, Purpura, Shore, Silver, etc.).

In the physiological model, drug action is described on the morphological (brain) level. Emphasis is placed on the interaction of psychotropic drugs with the function of the morphological substrate of the brain stem reticular formation, hypothalamic structures, limbic lobe, and neocortex (Berger, Bradley, Fields, Garattini, Ghatts, Hernandez-Peon, Himwich, Pennes, Streeker, Waelsch, etc.).

A comprehensive behavioral model of drug action was presented by Eysenck (1957). According to this model, human beings differ with respect to the speed with which excitation and inhibition are produced or dissipated and also with respect to the strength of the excitation and inhibition. As a second postulate, Eysenck stated that individuals in whom excitatory potential is weak are predisposed to develop extroverted patterns of behavior or hysterical-psychopathic disorders, while those in whom the excitatory potential is strong and generated quickly are predisposed to develop introverted patterns of behavior and dysthymic disorders. Applying this to drug action, Eysenck pointed out that (*a*) depressant drugs produce a decrease in the rate of conditioning, increase cortical inhibition, decrease cortical excitation, and produce extroverted behavioral patterns or an increase in hysterical and a decrease in dysthymic symptoms; (*b*) stimulant drugs produce an increase in the rate of conditioning, decrease cortical inhibition, increase cortical excitation, and produce introverted behavioral patterns or an increase in dysthymic and a decrease in hysterical symptoms.

Eysenck's theory was supported by his collaborators (Casey, Franks, Holland, etc.) in experimental studies on the effects of drugs (amylobaritone and amphetamine) on continuous work performance and visual aftereffects. Shagass and his collaborators (Jones, Mihalik, Naiman), using an electrophysiological procedure (Shagass' sedation threshold), came independently to results in favor of Eysenck's hypothesis. Shagass found that extroverts (psychopaths and hysterics) whose cortex is in a relatively inhibited state required relatively little of sodium amylobarbitone (depressant) before reaching the critical sedation point (low sedation threshold), while introverts (reactive depressives and obsessives) required relatively much before reaching the same critical sedation point (high sedation threshold).

In the clinical model, drug action is described in accordance with therapeutic implications. A comprehensive clinical model was proposed by Lehmann (1960). According to Lehmann, drug action is clinically characterized by the effects of the compounds on the psychological parameters of arousal, affect, or mental integration. Drugs that primarily influence the manifestations of the psychological parameter of arousal are the stimulants (trimethylxanthine, dextroamphetamine, methylphenidate, etc.) and the sedatives (bromides, barbiturates, etc.).

Drugs that have a facilitating effect on the psychological parameter of affect are the antidepressants (iminodibenzyls and monoamineoxidase inhibitors) and compounds that are helpful in apathy (phenothiazines with a piperidine or piperazine ring on the side chain). On the other side of this psychological parameter there are drugs with inhibitory properties: the minor tranquilizers (i.e., meprobamate, chlordiazepoxide, hydroxyphenamate, etc.), the major tranquilizers (phenothiazines, thioxanthenes, butyrophenones, rauwolfia alkaloids, etc.), and compounds with strong anti-manic effect (thioproperazine, reserpine, methyldopa, lithium, etc.).

Drugs whose clinical action is primarily upon mental integration are the psychotomimetics and the antipsychotic agents. Psychotomimetic drugs are chemicals (lysergic acid diethylamide, phenylethylamines, idolealkylamines, piperidylbenzilate-esters, phenilcyclohexyl piperidine, etc.) that induce mental derangement with a concomitant state resembling the psychoses. On the other hand, antipsychotics are drugs (phenothiazines, thioxanthenes, butyrophenones, rauwolfias, benzoquinolizines, etc.) that counteract specific psychotic symptoms based on mental disintegration or pathological integrations, such as delusions, hallucinations, etc.

The effects of psychotropic drugs with conditional reflex test procedures were studied by a great number of authors (Alexander, Alpern, Astrup, Balonov, Ban, Bridger, Faddeyeva, Finkelstein, Franks, Gantt, Gastaut, Gliedman, Hunt, Ivanov-Smolensky, Jenney, Jus, Kamirsky, Kerenyi, Laverty, Pfeiffer, Rajeva, Savchuk, Shumilina, Solyom, Taranskaya, Teitelbaum, etc.). Important findings were that the effect of the same drug differs when given in a single dose and when continuously administered, and also when given to normal subjects and to patients with definite psychopathology. Thus, for example, meprobamate, a minor tranquilizer, induces in normals "an inhibitory state in which reduction and dedifferentiation of the plethysmographic responses and paradoxical hypersynchrony of the electro-cerebral alerting responses" is manifest

(Astrup). The same drug in abnormal mental states promotes differentiation by reducing excitatory phenomena, including the paradoxical hypersynchrony of the electrocerebral alerting responses and the inhibitory generalizations (in neurotic depressions).

Similar findings were obtained with antipsychotic and antidepressant drugs, which, in a single dose administered to normals, instead of affecting the psychological parameter of mental integration or affect, respectively, lowered the level of arousal and produced inhibitory phenomena.

The effects of drugs on conditional reflex functions are presented schematically in the following paragraphs.

Stimulants, if administered in a single dose to normals, increase the strength of the unconditional reflex and decrease reaction time. A relatively larger number of stimulations is required to extinguish the orienting reflex, and a relatively smaller number of associated administrations of the conditional stimulus and unconditional stimulus to establish the conditional reflex. Similarly, the number of stimuli needed before differentiation takes place, secondary conditional reflex is formed, etc., decreases. The number of stimulations required from the extinction of the conditional reflex to the occurrence of the first EEG sign of sleep increases in direct proportion to the dosage administered. The transmission function from the first to the second signal system is facilitated, together with a decreased word association time, without qualitative change in the responses.

Sedatives, if administered in a single dose to normals, decrease the strength of the unconditional reflex and increase reaction time. Relatively fewer stimulations are required to extinguish the orienting reflex, and relatively more associated administrations of the conditional stimulus and unconditional stimulus to establish the conditional reflex; similarly, the number of stimuli needed before differentiation takes place or secondary conditional reflex is formed, etc. There is no qualitative alteration induced by sedatives in the transmission function from the first to the second signal system or in second signal system functions. There is a quantitatively measurable decrease in the transmission functions, with an increase in word association time.

Antidepressants, if chronically administered to depressed patients, have a normalizing effect on conditional reflex functions. This parallels the clinical improvement. The reaction time of the unconditional reflex decreases, while the strength of the response increases. Extinction rate of the orienting reflex increases to the normal range. Conditioning ability, differentiation, secondary conditional reflex formation, etc., improve (faster) during successful treatment. Sleep inhibition develops faster. The transmission from the first to the second signal system becomes prompter, and word association time shorter. There is also a normalization of verbal responses.

Depressants, if chronically administered to manic patients, have a normalizing effect on conditional reflex functions parallel with the clinical improvement. The reaction time of the unconditional reflex increases, and, respectively, the strength of the reactions decreases. Extinction rate of the orienting reflex decreases to the normal range. Conditioning ability, differentiation, secondary conditional reflex formation, etc., improves (slower). Sleep inhibition develops faster. There is also a normalization of verbal responses.

Psychotomimetics, if administered in a single dose to normals, do not always affect unconditional reflexes. The persistence of the orienting reflex increases; conditioning ability decreases; delayed and trace reflex formation becomes impaired. The transmission from the first to the second signal system decreases, word association time becomes longer, and there is also a shift from the higher-level responses to transient and primitive responses.

Antipsychotics, if chronically administered to schizophrenic patients, have a normalizing effect on conditional reflex functions. The persistence of the orienting reflex decreases. Conditioning ability, secondary conditional reflex, delayed and trace reflex formation improve. Generalization becomes more limited, and differentiation more accurate. The impairment of transmission functions from the first to the second signal system is counteracted by successful treatment; word association time decreases and there is a shift from the primitive and transient to higher responses.

In summary, psychotherapy and behavior therapy remain within the limits of conditioning theory—that is, information of overt behavior and neurophysiology—while pharmacotherapy serves to open new routes from neurophysiology to neurochemistry.

PART FIVE

*Critical
Evaluation*

11

CRITICAL EVALUATION

FEW SCIENTIFIC DATA remain valid if isolated from the philosophical stream that bore them, from the social setting where they were elaborated, and from the instrumentation that characterized the research of the period in which they originated. Pavlov's contribution, the introduction of the method of conditioning and the recognition of the implications of the conditional reflex, is among those which do. Fulton's statement that "Pavlov was one of the five or six individuals of the last generation who caused mankind to think in new terms; like Freud, he created a new horizon, but, unlike Freud, he seemed wholly objective in his mode of collecting scientific data" is now generally accepted.

Among contemporary intellectuals, acceptance of Pavlov's concept varied. Shaw, for example, considered Pavlov the biggest fool he had read about and remarked that "any policeman can tell that much about the dog," while Wells believed that "Pavlov's fame will grow with the ages." Similarly, the contemporary scientist's impression was best expressed by Sherrington, who remarked to a fellow physiologist after hearing Pavlov, "his observations are most brilliant but his deductions leave me cold."

BEHAVIORAL OBSERVATIONS

A critical evaluation of Pavlov's work with all its ramifications in a present-day scientific frame of reference has to be based on a comprehensive understanding of closely interrelated scientific disciplines.

Pavlov's work was grounded on the results of experiments

described in chapter 2 of this book, "Behavioral Observations."
Underlying his interpretation of these data was the assumption
that afferent activity at one point in the cortex and efferent
activity at another point, approximately at the same time,
are all that is needed to establish a sensory-motor connection
and that all behavior is determined by such conditioned connections. Furthermore, Pavlov assumed that all acts at the
time of a particular stimulation would be associated with the
stimulus and that the most frequently occurring would be
the most strongly associated. Hebb criticizes both these as-
sumptions. In the learning situation, Hebb points out, in
which several acts are possible, but only one rewarded, mistakes occur frequently. Often the same mistake is repeated
more frequently than the correct behavior. However the
mistakes vanish and leave only the correct responses. Since,
according to Pavlov, inhibition leads directly to sleep and
since repeated mistakes, according to Hebb, do not make the
animal drowsy but, on the contrary, often are followed by
increased activities, he concludes that the fact that the act
which occurred more frequently is forgotten cannot be ascribed
to inhibition.

Hebb's initial failure to confirm Pavlovian conditioning in
some of the learning situations does not invalidate Pavlov's
findings. On the other hand, it points to the fact that the
classical conditioning model cannot be schematically applied
in learning. Hebb clearly accepts conditioning, the preceding
coincidence of a conditional stimulus with an unconditional
stimulus, in that order, as the basis of learning; what he says
is that in some learning a third, motivational factor also
becomes important. When this motivational factor becomes
important, a different situation from the Pavlovian one sets in,
which follows different functional patterns. This three-dimen-
sional conception as an extension of the two-dimensional
Pavlovian, appeared first in the work of Konorski, who opposes
"instrumental conditioning" to the classical conditioning
method.

The same was expressed in Hull's modern learning–reinforcement theory, opposed to contiguity theories. Schlosberg

in his two-factor theory recognized the importance of both (classical conditioning versus instrumental conditioning and contiguity versus reinforcement theory) and considered them applicable to different functions (autonomic or skeleto-muscular, respectively), as did Skinner, who described the functional patterns of instrumental operant conditioning. The free operant conditioning method as applied by Lindsley extended its scope to include the conditional reflex in behavioral science.

PAVLOV'S BRAIN MODEL

Descartes' idea of *l'homme machine* was revived by Pavlov. He considered that "man is a system, a machine like every other system in nature, subject to the laws of all nature." As did Starling, Cannon, McDougall, and others, Pavlov recognized that adaptive behavior is equivalent to the behavior of a stable system, and he expressed the notion that "every material system can exist as an entity only as long as its internal forces, attractions, cohesions, etc., balance the external forces acting upon it." He claimed that "this is true for an ordinary stone just as much as for the most complex substance and its truth should be recognized also for the animal organism."

After many years of silence the concept of *l'homme machine,* and together with it Pavlov's brain model, were revived within the framework of cybernetics. Shannon demonstrated that a great number of behavior patterns could be produced artificially by a machine; furthermore, he showed that this could be done in an infinite variety of ways. Since Shannon's exposition several psychophysical models have been developed, some of them, like Ashby's, Walter's, and Uttley's, have used the conditional reflex as their basic function.

The use of these miniature models appeared to be a valuable exploratory method in the study of the functioning of the brain, which otherwise "can be explored only with great technical difficulty."

On the basis of this knowledge Ashby described Pavlov's brain model as a complex system that contains a number of parts or subfunctions. He considered Pavlov's model a multistage system in which the whole reaction is based on step functions, one activating the other in a chain. In this type of "machine" the natures of stimuli are to be determined in advance. But in the human mind functional circuits and feedbacks are also present, which Pavlov omitted from his model and which (according to Ashby) allow a greater variability of possible responses and protect against disorganization by new stimuli.

NEUROPHYSIOLOGICAL BASIS OF CONDITIONING

Conditioning is a behavioral method, and Pavlov assumed that there exists in the central nervous system a step-by-step representation of the various patterns of observable human behavior. Experiments by other investigators applying other methods contradicted Pavlov's inferences; for instance, strychninization revealed an entirely different kind of cortical organization from that which Pavlov had assumed (Hilgard and Marquis).

It was not before the extension of neurophysiology through electrophysiological instrumentation that Pavlov's neurophysiological concepts could be exposed to direct investigation. Although Pavlov himself became acquainted with the new instrumentation in Walter's laboratories, he did not apply electroencephalography in his own experiments.

The first comprehensive neurophysiological theory on conditioning by electrophysiological means was presented by Gastaut, who correlated his findings with those of Moruzzi and Magoun, Jasper, and Eccles. Since Gastaut's work, further contributions have been made in the field with microelectrode and electron-microscopic instrumentation. By these studies a great number of Pavlov's neurophysiological concepts have been disproved, among them the dominant role of the cerebral cortex in conditional reflex formation (Hernandez-Peon, etc.), but it also became increasingly evident that the Pavlovian conditional reflex and its functional patterns do exist, even if related to structures different from those he had assumed. In spite of considerable effort, generally accepted functional localizations of these patterns have not yet been established.

Fulton, in his book *The Physiology of the Nervous System,* pointed out that the conditioning method is feasible for the purpose of analyzing physiologically the intricate and unstable patterns characteristic of the individual's behavior. He stated also that "modifications and new applications of Pavlov's technique have led to rapid advances in the physiological analysis of behavior." However, with the accumulation of knowledge, some weak and controversial concepts of Pavlovian psychopathology were illuminated. Eysenck, in discussing Pavlov's typology, pointed out that Pavlov attempted to deduce from observations made on dogs the three main factors that determine human behavior and that are neurophysiologically based on the strength of the basic nervous processes, on the equilibrium of these processes, and on their mobility. Eysenck drew attention to the fact that Pavlov was thinking of human types as a homogeneous, non-continuous group. As he expressed it:

> The possible variations of the basic properties of the nervous system as well as the possible combinations of these variations determine the type of the nervous system; which as calculated amounts at least to twenty-four. But life shows that the actual number is considerably smaller; we distinguish between four types which are particularly distinct and strongly pronounced, and, what is most important, differ in their adaptability to the external environment and their resistibility to morbific agents.

Eysenck discards Pavlov's typology and offers instead a dimensional approach stressing the existence of continuity in the non-homogeneous group. Pushing further this concept, Eysenck pointed out that identifying the sanguine type with the extreme predominance of the excitatory process and the

melancholic type with the extreme predominance of the inhibitory process is contradictory in Pavlov's conceptions. According to Pavlov, neurosis in dogs is manifested either by
the predominance of excitation or by a predominance of
inhibition. These he compared to the two best-known forms
of the neuroses at the time. Thus Pavlov seemed to consider
that the neurasthenic type of neurosis is based on the weakness of the basic process of inhibition with a relative exaggeration of the basic process of excitation and is related to the
sanguine temperamental type, while the hysterical type of
neurosis is based on the weakness of the basic process of
excitation with the relative exaggeration of the basic process
of inhibition and is related to the melancholic temperamental
type.

Discarding at first Pavlov's typology, Eysenck disagreed
also with this conception and pointed out that, in contrast to
the theoretical formulation, it is the hysteric and not the
neurasthenic who is lively and sanguine, and it is the neurasthenic and not the hysteric who is cowardly and melancholic.

On the basis of a systematic appraisal of Pavlov's work
Eysenck considered that "Pavlov does not in fact present us
with a proper theory of personality derived from his conditioning experiments, but is more concerned to point out
certain analogies and possible methods of research in the
fields of normal and abnormal personality."

Pavlovian psychopathology and the classical Pavlovian approach to psychiatry is, in general, a teleological one. It is a
dynamic and descriptive psychiatry based on similarities observed during experimentation conducted on animals.

The approach is teleological, since it purposefully selects
evidence from the experimental results that fit into the contemporary psychiatric frame of reference expressed by Janet,
Meyer, Kretschmer, and others; Pavlov did not even attempt
to give any different conception of the psychopathological
manifestations. What Pavlov did was to offer a behaviorally
based understanding of the symptoms.

The dynamic principle of Pavlov's psychiatry is also related
to the contemporary views in the field. The conception that

psychiatric illness is the result of an interaction between the organism and its surroundings gained increasing acceptance in psychiatry at that time. The idea of continuity from the normal to the pathological is expressed by Pavlov in the statement that pathological variations are manifested in different hypnotic states. In other words, the same "symptoms" are present in different stages of normal sleep that are dominant in pathological (neurotic or psychotic) conditions. This immediately restricted Pavlov's psychiatry, even from a descriptive point of view. Out of the multitude of described variations elaborated by Bleuler's school on Kraepelin's solid basis, Pavlov preserved only those few that fitted into his conceptual framework. He restricted description to the well-known variations observed in his experimentation.

The major handicap of Pavlovian general and clinical psychopathology lies in the fact that it was based solely on animal experiments, applied schematically but analogously and lacking verification in humans.

FROM ANIMAL EXPERIMENTS TO HUMAN TEST PROCEDURES

Much of post-Pavlovian psychiatry has been characterized by an experimental approach. It was basically an attempt to correlate psychopathology with quantifiable laboratory findings. There was no major methodological development; only technical changes were made. Pavlov's experiments were replicated by using different conditioning techniques applicable to humans. Among these techniques the autonomic GSR and plethysmography, the semiautonomic, semivoluntary eyelid closure technique, and the voluntary skeletomuscular hand-withdrawal techniques, etc., were technically revised so that they could contribute to psychiatric knowledge. Although the techniques were revised and some of them highly developed, there was no general agreement in experimental design and interpretation of the findings, to the extent that, for example, in GSR conditioning some workers used an electroshock as the unconditional stimulus and tone as the conditional stimulus, and others the same tone as the unconditional stimulus. Because of the divergence in experimental design, contradictory findings were often presented by different workers. On the other hand, in this post-Pavlovian era the experimental method of conditioning was introduced into the clinical field and statistical means were applied in the evaluation of conditioning results.

An important finding in this era was the realization that the conditional reflex is not a duplicate of the unconditional reflex but is something new (Hilgard and Marquis, Zener, etc.). This was based on the observation that the dog whose food response was conditioned to hearing a bell is salivating to the auditory conditional stimulus but is not chewing and swallowing until food shows up. According to the classical Pavlovian hypothesis, the conditional stimulus is supposed to set up connections with *all* the following effector activity, which means also with eating movement and not just with salivary secretion. Since the dog's response is restricted to salivation, the Pavlovian classical conditioning model is also restricted in general to autonomic activity. The skeletomuscular, voluntary component, as, for example, the chewing movement, follows a different pattern, in which a third factor, motivation, comes into force (Konorski, Hull, Skinner, etc.). Thus, if the material placed in the mouth is tasty and edible, the activity that is initiated, besides salivary secretion, is chewing and swallowing, while if it is inedible, a defensive reaction becomes manifest in the action of spitting. Since the importance of voluntary activity increases with phylo- and ontogenetic development, the implications of classical conditioning in the understanding of human behavior proportionately diminishes.

CONDITIONING IN PSYCHIATRY

The neo-Pavlovian era is characterized by the physiological approach. It is based on correlations between neurophysiological findings and psychic symptoms, between pathophysiology and psychopathology. The growing amount of information obtained by psychopharmacological means is significant in this era.

The extension of the behavioral conditional reflex method with the physiological electroencephalographic method brought forth new findings, and the correlation of these with the psychopharmacological results led to newer concepts. Through these new methods, further evidence was given that a simultaneous afferent and efferent "activity" is not always sufficient for conditional reflex formation (Loucks). This neurophysiological evidence supports the behavioral findings that in the formation of the voluntary skeletomuscular conditional reflex a third motivational factor plays an important role.

Hovland pointed out that irradiation, which Pavlov assumed to be the basis of stimulus generalization, does not provide a sufficient basis for this function, and Loucks revealed that Pavlov's data disagree with his theoretical formulation of a slow irradiation of the basic processes of excitation and inhibition across the cortex.

While Pavlov's deductions became less acceptable in the neurophysiological neo–Pavlovian era, Pavlov's conditional reflex method became an increasingly valuable tool for the study of physiologically based psychic functions through behavioral manifestations. The orienting reflex behavior became an indicator of the arousal function of the brain stem reticular formation, correlated with the level of awareness and attention; the simple conditional reflex behavior became correlated with the sensory-emotional (relational) limbic lobe, hypothalamic activity, and the more complex conditional reflex phenomena, such as differentiation, etc., with sensory-motor (volitional) highly integrated cortical functions.

There are indications that neurotic disorders primarily affect the orienting reflex, becoming manifest in extremely high or extremely low degrees of arousal, while different psychotic conditions interfere with differentiation, delayed reflex formation, etc., that is, with the integrative functions. There are also indications that drugs that have only sedative or stimulating properties are ineffective in psychotic conditions when disintegration or pathological integration prevails, while so-called antipsychotic agents (phenothiazines, thioxanthenes, butyrophenones, benzoquinolizines) are therapeutic in such cases.

In the course of the neurophysiological development Pavlov's brain model, which is based on the continuous interplay of the two basic nervous processes of excitation and inhibition, their irradiation and concentration, became unacceptable for scientific validation. Not so the conditional reflex and related phenomena, which were given new neurophysiological formulations.

Pavlov, of course, had never pretended that his own observations or method would reveal the final answers to all "nervous" phenomena, but he believed that only a study of the physicochemical processes taking place in nerve tissue would give a real theory of all nervous phenomena and that the phases of these processes would provide us with a full understanding of all the external manifestations of the nervous activity, their consecutiveness and their interrelations.

While the work based on the method of conditioning was coming close to completion and gaining acceptance with the clinician, in research a chemical and pharmacological orientation and a new psychopharmacological methodology was gaining increasing importance. This new method has within a few years contributed more to psychiatric medical therapy than has any other method or approach in the past.

BIBLIOGRAPHY

ACKNER, B. 1956. Emotions and the peripheral vasomotor system. *J. Psychosom. Res.*, 1: 3.

ADAMS, D. K. 1937. Note on method. *Psychol. Rev.*, 44: 212.

ADRIAN, E. D. 1934. Electrical activity of the nervous system. *Arch. Neurol. Psychiat.*, 32: 1125.

———. 1936. The spread of activity in the cerebral cortex. *J. Physiol.*, 88: 127.

ADRIAN, E. D., and MATTHEWS, B. H. C. 1934. The Berger rhythm: potential changes from the occipital lobes in man. *Brain*, 57: 355.

ALBE-FESSARD, D., and GILLETT, E. 1958. Interaction au niveau du centre médian entre des influx, d'origine somesthésique et d'origine corticale; activités unitaires. *J. Physiol.* (Paris), 50: 108.

ALBE-FESSARD, D., OSWALDO-CRUZ, E., and ROCHA-MIRANDA, C. E. 1958. Convergence vers le noyau caudé de signaux d'origines corticales et hétérosensorielles, étude unitaire de leurs interactions. *J. Physiol.* (Paris), 50: 105.

ALBE-FESSARD, D., and ROUGEUL, A. 1956. Relais thalamiques d'afférences somesthésiques aboutissant à certaines régions localisées du cortex associatif du chat. *J. Physiol.* (Paris), 48: 370.

———. 1958. Activités d'origine somesthésique évoquées sur le cortex non-spécifique du chat anesthésié au chloralose: rôle du cerveau médian du thalamus. *Electroencephalog. Clin. Neurophysiol.*, 10: 131.

ALDRICH, C. A. 1928. A new test for hearing in the new born: the conditioned reflex. *Amer. J. Dis. Child.*, 35: 33.

ALEXANDER, L. 1958. Apparatus and method for the study of conditional reflexes in man. *Arch. Neurol. Psychiat.*, 80: 629.

ALEXANDER, L., and LIPSETT, S. 1959. Effect of amine oxidase inhibitors on the conditioned PGR in man. *Dis. Nerv. Syst.*, 20: 33.

ALLEN, W. F. 1937. Olfactory and trigeminal conditioned reflexes in dogs. *Amer. J. Physiol.*, 118: 532.

———. 1938. Relationship of the conditioned olfactory foreleg response to the motor centers of the brain. *Ibid.*, 121: 657.

ALPERN, E. B., FINKELSTEIN, N., and GANTT, W. H. 1941. Effect of amphetamine sulfate on the nervous activity of dogs. *Amer. J. Physiol.*, 133: 195.

———. 1943. Effect of amphetamine (benzedrine) sulfate upon higher nervous activity. I. Animal experiments. *Bull. Johns Hopkins Hosp.*, 73: 287.

———. 1945. Effect of amphetamine (benzedrine) sulfate upon higher nervous activity compared with alcohol. II. Human experiments. *Ibid.*, 76: 61.

ANOKHIN, P. K. 1957. The significance of the reticular formation for various forms of higher nervous activity. *J. Physiol.*, 43: 1072.

———. 1960. On the specific action of the reticular formation on the cerebral cortex. *Electroencephalog. Clin. Neurophysiol.*, Suppl. 13, p. 257.

ANREP, G. V. 1920. Pitch discrimination in the dog. *J. Physiol.*, 53: 367.

———. 1923. The irradiation of conditioned reflexes. *Proc. Roy. Soc.*, 94: 404.

APTER, I. M. 1957. Comparisons of the effects of ECT, camphor and a combination of ECT and prolonged sleep on the higher nervous activity of dogs. (Rus.) *Z. Nevropat. Psikhiat. (Korsakoff)*, Suppl. 57, p. 89.

———. 1958. The dynamics of the higher nervous activity of neurasthenic patients during treatment. *Ibid.*, 58: 1321.

ARDUINI, A., and ARDUINI, M. G. 1954. Effect of drugs and metabolic alterations on brain stem arousal mechanism. *J. Pharmacol. Exp. Ther.*, 110: 76.

ARNOLD, W. J. 1945. An exploratory investigation of primary response generalization. *J. Comp. Psychol.*, 38: 87.

———. 1947. Simple reaction chains and their integration. I. Homogeneous chaining with terminal reinforcement. *J. Comp. Physiol. Psychol.*, 40: 349.

———. 1947. Simple reaction chains and their integration. II. Heterogeneous chaining with terminal reinforcement. *Ibid.*, p. 427.

———. 1948. Simple reaction chains and their integration. III. Heterogeneous chaining with serial reinforcement. *Ibid.*, 41: 1.

———. 1951. Simple reaction chains and their integration. IV. Homogeneous chaining with serial reinforcement. *Ibid.*, 44: 276.

ARTEMYEV, V. V. 1956. Some electrophysiological aspects of the mechanism of conditioned reflexes. (Rus.) *Publ. Pavlov Fiziol. Inst.*, 5: 110.

ASCHAFFENBURG, G. 1896. Experimentelle Studien über Associationen: die Associationen im normalen Zustande. *Psychol. Arb.*, 1: 209.

———. 1904. Experimentelle Studien über Associationen: die Ideenflucht. *Ibid.*, 4: 235.

ASHBY, W. R. 1950. A new mechanism which shows simple conditioning. *J. Psychol.*, 29: 343.

———. 1954. *Design for a Brain.* Wiley.

ASTRUP, C. 1955. Untersuchungen mit der Assoziationsmethode über Störungen im zweiten Signalsystem bei verschiedenen psychopathologischen Zustanden. *Psychiat. Neurol. Med. Psychol.*, 7: 326.

―――. 1956. Erfahrungen mit verschiedenen bedingtreflektorischen Untersuchungmethoden an Neurotikern. *Ibid.*, 8: 161.

―――. 1957. Experimentelle Untersuchungen über die Störungen der höheren Nerventätigkeit bei akuten und subchronischen Schizophrenen. *Ibid.*, 9: 33.

―――. 1957. Experimentelle Untersuchungen über die Störungen der höheren Nerventätigkeit bei Defektschizophrenen. *Ibid.*, p. 9.

―――. 1957. Experimentelle Untersuchungen über die Störungen der höheren Nerventätigkeit bei Manisch-Depressiven Psychosen. *Ibid.*, p. 369.

―――. 1957. Experimentelle Untersuchungen über die Störungen der höheren Nerventätigkeit bei Oligophrenen. *Ibid.*, p. 377.

―――. 1957. Experimentelle Untersuchungen über die Störungen der höheren Nerventätigkeit bei Organisch Dementen und Organischen Psychosen. *Ibid.*, p. 380.

―――. 1957. Experimentelle Untersuchungen über die Störungen der höheren Nerventätigkeit bei Reaktiven (psychogenen) Psychosen. *Ibid.*, p. 373.

―――. 1958. Klinische-experimentelle Untersuchungen bei verschiedenen Formen von Schizophrenie. *Ibid.*, 10: 355.

―――. 1959. The effects of ataraxic drugs on schizophrenic subgroups related to experimental findings. *Acta Psychiat. Scand.*, Suppl., 136: 388.

―――. 1962. *Schizophrenia: Conditional Reflex Studies.* Charles C Thomas.

BABINSKI, M. J. 1901. Definition of hysteria. *Rev. Neurol.*, 9: 138.

BABKIN, B. P. 1951. *Pavlov: A Biography.* Gollancz.

BALONOV, L. J. 1958. The "sore points" of the cerebral cortex connected with pathological changes of cardiac activity. (Rus.) *Tez. 18. Sov. Probl. Vyss. Nerv. Dejat.*, 2: 39.

BALONOV, L. J., LICHKO, A. E., and TRAUGOTT, N. N. 1957. Oppression and restoration of the higher nervous activity in some pathological conditions. (Rus.) *Z. Vyss. Nerv. Dejat. Pavlova* 7: 335.

BALONOV, L. J., and TRAUGOTT, N. N. 1958. Disturbances of the higher nervous activity in various depressive states. (Rus.) *Tez. 18 Sov. Probl. Vyss. Nerv. Dejat.*, 2: 36.

BARANOV, V. G. 1955. Data about the higher nervous activity in thyreotoxicosis and hypothyreosis (Rus.) *Z. Vyss. Nerv. Dejat. Pavlova*, 5: 336.

BARLOW, J. A. 1956. Secondary motivation through classical conditioning: a reconsideration of the nature of backward conditioning. *Psychol. Rev.*, 63: 406.

BARLOW, J. S. 1957. An electronic method for detecting evoked responses of the brain and for reproducing their average waveforms. *Electroencephalog. Clin. Neurophysiol.*, 9: 340.

BARLOW, J. S., and BRAZIER, M. A. B. 1954. A note on a correlator for electroencephalographic work. *Electroencephalog. Clin. Neurophysiol.*, 6: 321.

BARNES, G. W. 1956. Conditioned stimulus intensity and temporal factors in spaced-trial classical conditioning. *J. Exp. Psychol.*, 51: 192.

BARNETT, C. D., and CANTOR, G. N. 1951. Discrimination set in defectives. *Amer. J. Ment. Defic.*, 62: 334.

BASKINA, N. F. 1953. Concerning peculiarities of the auditory analyser during auditory hallucinations. (Rus.) *Z. Nevropat. Psikhiat. (Korsakoff)*, 53: 840.

BASS, B. 1958. Gradients in response percentages as indices of non-spatial generalization. *J. Exp. Psychol.*, 56: 278.

BASS, M. J., and HULL, C. L. 1934. The irradiation of a tactile conditioned reflex in man. *J. Comp. Psychol.*, 17: 47.

BECK, E. C., and DOTY, R. W. 1957. Conditioned flexion reflexes acquired during combined catelepsy and de-efferentation. *J. Comp. Physiol. Psychol.*, 50: 211.

BECK, E. C., DOTY, R. W., and KOOI, K. A. 1958. Electrocortical reactions associated with conditioned flexion reflexes. *Electroencephalog. Clin. Neurophysiol.*, 10: 279.

BEHAN, R. A. 1953. Expectancies and Hullian theory. *Psychol. Rev.*, 60: 252.

BEIER, D. G. 1940. Conditioning cardiovascular responses and suggestion for the treatment of cardiac neurosis. *J. Exp. Psychol.*, 27: 311.

BEKHTEREV, V. M. 1913. *La Psychologie Objective*. Alcan.

———. 1913. *Objektive Psychologie oder Psychoreflexologie: die Lehre von der Assoziations-Reflexen*. Teubner.

———. 1928. *General Principles of Human Reflexology*. Translated by E. and W. MURPHY. International Publishers.

BENDER, L., and SCHILDER, P. 1930. Unconditioned and conditioned reactions to pain in schizophrenia. *Amer. J. Psychiat.*, 87: 365.

BERGMAN, G. 1956. The contribution of John B. Watson. *Psychol. Rev.*, 63: 265.

BERITASHVILI, I. S. 1956. The morphological and physiological bases of temporary connections in the cerebral cortex. (Rus.) *Publ. Beritashvili Inst. Fiziol.*, 10: 3.

BERITOV, I. S. 1924. On the fundamental nervous process in the cortex of the cerebral hemispheres. *Brain*, 47: 109.

BERNHAUT, M., GELLHORN, E., and RASMUSSEN, A. T. 1953. Experimental contributions to the problem of consciousness. *J. Neurophysiol.*, 16: 21.

BERNSTEIN, A. L. 1934. Temporal factors in the formation of conditioned eyelid reactions in human subjects. *J. Gen. Psychol.*, 10: 173.

BERSH, P. J., SCHOENFELD, W. N., and NOTTERMAN, J. M. 1953. The effect upon heart-rate conditioning of randomly varying the interval between conditioned and unconditioned stimuli. *Proc. Nat. Acad. Sci.*, 39: 563.

BINDRA, D., *et al.* 1955. On the relation between anxiety and conditioning. *Can. J. Psychol.*, 9: 1.

BIRNBAUM, K. 1912. Uber den Einfluss von Gefühlsfaktoren auf die Assoziationen. *Mschr. Psychiat. Neurol.*, 32: 95.

BITTERMAN, M. E. 1957. Book review of Behavior Therapy and Conditioning by K. W. SPENCE. *Amer. J. Psychol.*, 70: 141.

BITTERMAN, M. E., FEDDERSON, W. E., and TYLER, D. W. 1953. Secondary reinforcement and the discrimination hypothesis. *Amer. J. Psychol.*, 66: 456.

BITTERMAN, M. E., and HOLTZMAN, W. H. 1952. Conditioning and extinction of the galvanic skin response as a function of anxiety. *J. Abnorm. Soc. Psychol.*, 47: 615.

BITTERMAN, M. E., REED, P., and KRAUSKOPF, J. 1952. The effect of the duration of the unconditioned stimulus upon conditioning and extinction. *Amer. J. Psychol.*, 65: 256.

BITTERMAN, M. E., and WODINSKY, J. 1953. Simultaneous and successive discrimination. *Psychol. Rev.*, 60: 371.

BLACK, A. H. 1958. The extinction of avoidance responses under curare-like drugs. *J. Comp. Physiol. Psychol.*, 51: 519.

BLAGOSKLONNAYA, Y. V., KALNINA, E. I., and PANINA, G. P. 1955. Some characteristics of the vascular reactions in neurasthenia. (Rus.) *Klin. Med.*, 33: 45.

BOGOSLOVSKI, A. I. 1937. An attempt at creating sensory conditioned reflexes in humans. *J. Exp. Psychol.*, 21: 403.

BONEAU, C. A. 1958. The interstimulus interval and the latency of the conditioned eyelid response. *J. Exp. Psychol.*, 56: 464.

BRADY, J. V. 1951. The effect of electro-convulsive shock on a conditioned emotional response: the permanence of the effect. *J. Comp. Physiol. Psychol.*, 44: 507.

———. 1952. The effect of electro-convulsive shock on a conditioned emotional response: the significance of the interval between the emotional conditioning and the electro-convulsive shock. *Ibid.*, 45: 9.

———. 1956. Emotional behavior and the nervous system. *Trans. N.Y. Acad. Sci.*, 18: 601.

———. 1957. A comparative approach to the evaluation of drug effects upon affective behavior. *Ann. N.Y. Acad. Sci.*, 64: 632.

BRADY, J V., and HUNT, H. F. 1951. A further demonstration of the effect of electro-convulsive shock on a conditional emotional response. *J. Comp. Physiol. Psychol.*, 44: 204.

———. 1955. An experimental approach to the analysis of emotional behaviour. *J. Psychol.*, 40: 313.

BRADY, J. V., HUNT, H. F., and GELLER, I. 1954. The effect of electro-convulsive shock on a conditional emotional response as a function of the temporal distribution of the treatments. *J. Comp. Physiol. Psychol.*, 47: 454.

BRADY, J. V., STEBBINS, W. C., and GALAMBOS, R. 1953. The effect of audiogenic convulsions on a conditioned emotional response. *J. Comp. Physiol. Psychol.*, 46: 363.

BRADY, J. V., STEBBINS, W. C., and HUNT, H. F. 1953. The effect of electro-convulsive shock (ECS) on a conditioned emotional response: the effect of additional ECS convulsions. *J. Comp. Physiol. Psychol.*, 46: 368.

BRAGIEL, R. M., and PERKINS, C. C., JR. 1954. Conditioned stimulus intensity and response speed. *J. Exp. Psychol.*, 47: 437.

BRAIN, H. 1958. The physiological basis of consciousness: a critical review. *Brain*, 81: 426.

BRAUN, H. W., and GEISELHART, R. 1959. Age differences in the acquisition and extinction of the conditioned eyelid response. *J. Exp. Psychol.*, 57: 386.

BRAZIER, M. A. B. (ed.). 1959. *The Central Nervous System and Behaviour: Transactions of the First Conference.* Josiah Macy Jr. Foundation.

————. 1959. *The Central Nervous System and Behaviour: Transactions of the Second Conference.* Josiah Macy Jr. Foundation.

————. 1960. *The Central Nervous System and Behaviour: Transactions of the Third Conference.* Josiah Macy Jr. Foundation.

BREGMAN, E. O. 1934. An attempt to modify the emotional attitudes of infants by the conditioned response technique. *J. Genet. Psychol.*, 45: 169.

BRIDGER, W. H., and GANTT, W. H. 1956. The effect of mescaline on differentiated conditional reflexes. *Amer. J. Psychiat.*, 113: 352.

BROGDEN, W. J. 1938. The unconditioned stimulus substitution in the conditioning process. *Amer. J. Physiol.*, 123: 24.

————. 1939. Higher order conditioning. *Amer J. Psychol.*, 52: 579.

————. 1939. Sensory preconditioning. *J. Exp Psychol.*, 25: 323.

————. 1939. The effect of frequency of reinforcement upon the level of conditioning. *J. Exp. Psychol.*, 24: 419.

————. 1939. Unconditioned stimulus substitution in the conditioning process. *Amer. J. Psychol.*, 52: 46.

————. 1940. Lateral cerebral dominance in the dog tested by the conditioning and extinction of forelimb flexion. *J. Gen. Psychol.*, 23: 387.

————. 1941. Effect of change in time of reinforcement in the maintenance of conditioned flexion responses in dogs. *J. Exp. Psychol.*, 29: 49.

————. 1942. Non-alimentary components in the food reinforcement of conditioned forelimb-flexion in dogs. *Ibid.*, 30: 325.

————. 1947. Sensory preconditioning of human subjects. *Ibid.*, 37: 527.

————. 1949. Acquisition and extinction of a conditioned response in dogs. *J. Comp. Physiol. Psychol.*, 42: 296.

————. 1950. Sensory conditioning measured by the facilitation of auditory acuity. *J. Exp. Psychol.*, 40: 512.

BROGDEN, W. J., and CULLER, E. 1936. Device for the motor conditioning of small animals. *Science*, 83: 269.

BROGDEN, W. J., and GANTT, W. H. 1937. Cerebellar conditioned reflexes. *Amer. J. Physiol.*, 119: 277.

————. 1942. Intraneural conditioning: cerebellar-conditioned reflexes. *Arch. Neurol. Psychiat.*, 48: 437.

BROGDEN, W. J., LIPMAN, E. A., and CULLER, E. 1938. The role of incentive in conditioning and extinction. *Amer. J. Psychol*, 51: 109.

BROMILEY, R. B. 1948. Conditioned responses in a dog after removal of the neocortex. *J. Comp. Physiol. Psychol.*, 41: 102.

BROTHERS, J. D., and WAROLEN, C. J. 1950. An analysis of the enzyme activity of the conditioned salivary response in human subjects. *Science*, 112: 751.

BROWN, C. C. 1957. Changes in avoidance conditioning following psychotherapeutic treatment. *J. Nerv. Ment. Dis.*, 125: 487.

BROWN, C C., RUDO, M., and GANTT, W. H. 1955. Autonomic responses to mecholyl and epinephrine injections in schizophrenic patients. *J. Pharmacol. Exp. Ther.*, 113: 8.

BROWN, J. S. 1939. A note on a temporal gradient of reinforcement. *J. Exp. Psychol.*, 25: 221.

BROWN, J. S., CLARKE, F. R., and STEIN, L. 1958. A new technique for studying spatial generalization with voluntary responses. *J. Exp. Psychol.*, 55: 359.

BROWN, J. S., and JACOBS, A. 1949. The role of fear in the motivation and acquisition of responses. *J. Exp. Psychol.*, 39: 747.

BROWN, J. S., KALISH, H. I., and FARBER, I. E. 1951. Conditioned fear as revealed by magnitude of startle response to an auditory stimulus. *J. Exp. Psychol.*, 41: 317.

BRUSH, F. R., BRUSH, L. S., and SOLOMON, R. L. 1955. Traumatic avoidance learning: the effects of CS-US interval with a delayed-conditioning procedure. *J. Comp. Physiol. Psychol.*, 48: 285.

BÜHLER, K. 1949. *The Mental Development of the Child.* Routledge & Kegan Paul.

BUMKE, O., and KEHRER, F. 1910. Plethysmographische Untersuchungen an Geisteskranken. *Arch. Psychiat. Nervenkr.*, 47: 945.

BURN, J. H., and HOBBS, H. 1958. A test for tranquilizing drugs. *Arch. Int. Pharmacodyn.*, 113: 290.

BURNHAM, W. H. 1917. Mental hygiene and the conditioned reflex. *J. Genet. Psychol.*, 24: 449.

BUSER, P. 1957. Activités de projection et d'association du néocortex cérebral des mammifères: activités d'association et d'élaboration: projections non-specifiques. *J. Physiol.* (Paris), 49: 589.

BUSER, P. and BORENSTEIN, P. 1956. Données sur la répartition des réponses sensorielles corticales (somesthésiques, visuelles, auditives) chez le chat curarisé non-anesthésié. *J. Physiol.* (Paris), 48: 419.

――――. 1957. Réponses corticales "secondaires" à la stimulation sensorielle chez le chat curarisé non-anesthésié. *Electroencephalog. Clin. Neurophysiol.*, Suppl., 6: 89.

――――. 1957. Suppression élective de réponses "associatives" par stimulation réticulaire chez le chat sous anesthésie profonde au chloralose. *J. Physiol.* (Paris), 49: 86.

BUSER, P., JOUVET, M., and HERNANDEZ-PEON, R. 1958. Modifications au cours du conditionnement chez le chat du cycle d'excitabilité au niveau de la réticulée mésencéphalique. *Acta Neurol. Latinoamer.*, 4: 268.

BUSER, P., and ROUGEUL, A. 1956. Réponses sensorielles corticales chez le chat en préparation chronique: leurs modifications lors de l'établissement de liaisons temporaires. *Rev. Neurol.*, 95: 501.

BYKOV, K. M. 1957. *The Cerebral Cortex and the Internal Organs.* Translated and edited by W. H. GANTT. Chemical Publishing Co.

CALKINS, M. W. 1892. A suggested classification of cases of association. *Philos. Rev.*, 1: 389.

CAMPBELL, A. A. 1938. The interrelations of two measures of conditioning in man. *J. Exp. Psychol.*, 22: 225.

CAMPBELL, A. A., and HILGARD, E. R. 1936. Individual differences in ease of conditioning. *J. Exp. Psychol.*, 19: 561.

CANTOR, E. 1911. Ergebnisse von Assoziation-versuchen mittels blossen Zurufs bei Schwachsinnigen. *Mschr. Psychiat. Neurol.*, 29: 335.

CAPALDI, E. J. 1958. The effect of different amounts of training on the resistance to extinction of different patterns of partially reinforced responses. *J. Comp. Physiol. Psychol.*, 51: 367.

CAPEHART, J., VINEY, W., and HULICKA, I. M. 1958. The effect of effort upon extinction. *J. Comp. Physiol. Psychol.*, 51: 505.

CARTER, L. F. 1941. Intensity of conditioned stimulus and rate of conditioning. *J. Exp. Psychol.*, 28: 481.

CASON, H. 1922. The conditioned eyelid reaction. *J. Exp. Psychol.*, 5: 1953.

――――. 1922. The conditioned pupillary reaction. *Ibid.*, p. 108.

――――. 1925. The conditioned reflex or conditioned response as a common activity of living organisms. *Psychol. Bull.*, 22: 445.

――――. 1925. The physical basis of the conditioned response. *Amer. J. Psychol.*, 36: 371.

――――. 1932. The pleasure-pain theory of learning. *Psychol. Rev.*, 39: 440.

————. 1933. Sensory conditioning. *J. Exp. Psychol.*, 16: 572.

————. 1934. Dr. Hilgard on the conditioned eyelid reaction. *Ibid.*, 17: 894.

————. 1934. The role of verbal activities in the conditioning of human subjects. *Psychol. Rev.*, 41: 563.

————. 1935. Backward conditioned eyelid reactions. *J. Exp. Psychol.*, 18: 599.

————. 1936. Sensory conditioning. *Ibid.*, 19: 572.

CASON, H., and KATCHER, N. 1931. An attempt to condition breathing and eyelid responses to a subliminal electric stimulus. *J. Exp. Psychol.*, 16: 831.

CHAMBERS, R. M., and FULLER, J. L. 1958. Conditioning of skin temperature changes in dogs. *J. Comp. Physiol. Psychol.*, 51: 223.

CHANG, H. T. 1950. The repetitive discharges of the cortico-thalamic reverberating circuit. *J. Neurophysiol.*, 13: 236.

————. 1951. Dendritic potential of cortical neurons produced by direct electrical stimulation of the cerebral cortex. *Ibid.*, 14: 1.

CHAPMAN, W. P. 1944. Measurements of pain sensitivity in normal control subjects and in psychoneurotic subjects. *Psychosom. Med.*, 6: 252.

CHERNACHEK, I. 1956. A study of the pathophysiology of hysterical symptoms by the method of conditional reflexes. (Rus.) *Z. Nevropat. Psikhiat. (Korsakoff)*, 56: 858.

CHEYMAN, I .M. 1957. The natural conditional reflexes of chronic alcoholics as signs of their treatment progress. (Rus.) *Z. Nevropat. Psikhiat. (Korsakoff)*, 57: 1235.

CHISTOVICH, A. S. 1949. The opinions of Pavlov on schizophrenia. (Rus.) *Nevropat. i Psikhiat.*, 18: 52.

————. 1952. Some data on the pathophysiological understanding of acute infectious psychoses. (Rus.) *Z. Vyss. Nerv. Dejat. Pavlova*, 2: 78.

————. 1955. The role of infections in the development of some mental disorders. (Rus.) *Z. Nevropat. Psikhiat. (Korsakoff)*, 55: 843.

CHURCH, R. M., BRUSH, F. R., and SOLOMON, R. L. 1956. Traumatic avoidance learning. The effects of CS-US interval with a delayed conditioning procedure in a free-responding situation. *J. Comp. Physiol. Psychol.*, 49: 301.

CLARKE, A. D. B. 1955. Motor and memory responses of neurotics and normals in the Luria association-motor technique. *Brit. J. Psychol.*, 46: 38.

COHEN, J. 1950. Observations on strictly simultaneous conditioned reflexes. *J. Comp. Physiol. Psychol.*, 43: 211.

COOK, L., and WEIDLEY, E. 1957. Behavioral effects of some psychopharmacological agents. *Ann. N.Y. Acad. Sci.*, 66: 740.

COOK, S. W. 1939. A survey of methods used to produce "experimental neurosis." *Amer. J. Psychiat.*, 95: 1259.

————. 1939. The production of "experimental neurosis" in the white rat. *Psychosom. Med.*, 1: 293.

Cook, S. W., and Harris, R. E. 1937. The verbal conditioning of the galvanic skin reflex. *J. Exp. Psychol.*, 21: 202.

Coombs, C. H. 1938. Adaptation of the galvanic response to auditory stimuli. *J. Exp. Psychol.*, 22: 244.

Cordeau, J. P., and Mancia, M. 1959. Evidence for the existence of an EEG synchronization mechanism originating in the lower brain stem. *Electroencephalog. Clin. Neurophysiol.*, 11: 551.

Corson, S. A., *et al.* 1961. Differential effects of meprobamate on conditioned renal and motor defence responses. *Biochem. Pharm.*, 8: 174.

Crasilneck, H. B., and McRanie, E. J. 1956. On the conditioning of the pupillary reflex. *J. Psychol.*, 42: 23.

Crisler, G. 1930. Salivation is unnecessary for the establishment of the salivary conditioned reflex induced by morphine. *Amer. J. Physiol.*, 94: 553.

Crown, S. 1947. A controlled association test as a measure of neuroticism. *J. Personality*, 16: 198.

Crum, J., Brown, W. L., and Bitterman, M. E. 1951. The effect of partial and delayed reinforcement on resistance to extinction. *Amer. J. Psychol.*, 64: 228.

Culler, E., Finch, G., and Girden, E. 1934. Apparatus for motor conditioning in cats. *Science*, 79: 525.

Culler, E., Finch, G., Girden, E., and Brogden, W. J. 1935. Measurements of acuity by the conditioned response techniques. *J. Gen. Psychol.*, 12: 223.

Culler, E., and Mettler, F. A. 1934. Conditioned behavior in a decorticate dog. *J. Comp. Psychol.*, 18: 291.

Darrow, C. W. 1947. Psychological and psychophysiological significance of the electroencephalogram. *Psychol. Rev.*, 54: 157.

Davis, H., *et al.* 1938. Human brain potentials during the onset of sleep. *J. Neurophysiol.*, 1: 24.

Delafresnaye, J. F., Fessard, A., Gerard, R. W., and Konorski, J. (eds.). 1961. *Brain Mechanism and Learning.* Charles C Thomas.

Delgado, J. M. R., Roberts, W. W., and Miller, N. E. 1954. Learning motivated by electrical stimulation of the brain. *Amer. J. Physiol.*, 179: 587.

Delgado, J. M. R., Rosvold, H. E., and Looney, E. 1956. Evoking conditioned fear by electrical stimulation of subcortical structures in the monkey brain. *J. Comp. Physiol. Psychol.*, 49: 373.

Dempsey, E. W., and Morison, R. S. 1942. The production of rhythmically recurrent cortical potentials after localized thalamic stimulation. *Amer. J. Physiol.*, 135: 293.

Dews, P. B. 1956. Modification by drugs of performances on simple schedules of positive reinforcement. *Ann N.Y. Acad. Sci.*, 65: 268.

Dmitriev, A. S. 1956. Contribution to the methods of studying higher nervous activity in man. (Rus.) *Z. Vyss. Nerv. Dejat. Pavlova*, 6: 906.

Dmitriev, L. I. 1958. The interactions of somatic and autonomic conditional and unconditional reactions in the stuporous form of catatonic schizophrenia. (Rus.) *Tr. Inst. Vyss. Nerv. Dejat. Ser. Patofiziol.*, 5: 21.

———. 1958. Studies of the combined activity of the cortical signalling systems in the stuporous form of catatonic schizophrenia. *Ibid.*, p. 38.

Dmitrieva, A. F. 1958. The higher nervous activity in various types of neurasthenia. (Rus.) *Tr. Inst. Fiziol. Im. I. P. Pavlov*, 7: 97.

Dmitrieva, A. F., *et al.* 1958. The determination of the type of higher nervous activity in patients with neuroses. (Rus.) *Tr. Inst. Fiziol. Im. I. P. Pavlov*, 7: 106.

Dobrzhanskaya, A. K. 1954. The cortical functions and the interaction of the signalling systems in the acute stage of schizophrenia. (Rus.) *Z. Vyss. Nerv. Dejat. Pavlova*, 4: 502.

Dollard, J., and Miller, N. E. 1950. *Personality and Psychotherapy.* McGraw-Hill.

Domino, E. F. 1955. A pharmacological analysis of the functional relationship between the brain stem arousal and diffuse thalamic projection system. *J. Pharmacol. Exp. Ther.*, 115: 449.

Doty, R. W., and Rutledge, L. T. 1959. Conditioned reflexes elicited by stimulation of partially isolated cerebral cortex. *Fed. Proc.*, 37: 18.

Doty, R. W., Rutledge, L. T., and Larsen, R. M. 1956. Conditioned reflexes established to electrical stimulation of cat cerebral cortex. *J. Neurophysiol.*, 19: 401.

Dumont, S., and Dell, P. 1958. Facilitations spécifiques et non-spécifiques des réponses visuelles corticales. *J. Physiol.* (Paris), 50: 261.

Durup, G., and Fessard, A. 1935. L'electroencephalogramme de l'homme. *Année Psychol.*, 36: 1.

Dworkin, L. 1939. Conditioning neuroses in dog and cat. *Psychosom. Med.* 1: 388.

Dykman, R. A., and Gantt, W. H. 1951. A comparative study of cardiac conditioned responses and motor conditioned responses in controlled "Stress" situations. *Amer. J. Physiol.*, 6: 263.

———. 1954. Blood pressure conditioned to pain. *Fed. Proc.*, 13: 127.

Dykman, R. A., and Shurrager, P. S. 1956. Successive and maintained conditioning in spinal carnivores. *J. Comp. Physiol. Psychol.*, 49: 27.

ECCLES, J. C. 1946. Synaptic potentials of motorneurons. *J. Neurophysiol.*, 9: 87.

————. 1953. *The Neurophysiological Basis of Mind*. Clarendon Press.

————. 1957. *The Physiology of Nerve Cells*. Johns Hopkins Press.

ECCLES, J. C., and RALL, W. 1951. Effects induced in a monosynaptic reflex path by its activation. *J. Neurophysiol.*, 14: 353.

EHRENFREUND, D. 1949. Effect of a secondary reinforcing agent in black-white discrimination. *J. Comp. Physiol. Psychol.*, 42: 1.

ELLISON, D. 1939. The concept of reflex reserve. *Psychol. Rev.*, 46: 566.

ELLISON, D. 1939. Spontaneous recovery of the galvanic skin response as a function of the recovery interval. *J. Exp. Psychol.*, 25: 586.

ENGLISH, H. B. 1929 Three cases of the "conditioned fear response." *J. Abnorm. Soc. Psychol.*, 24: 221.

EROFEEVA, M. 1916. Contributions à l'étude des reflexes conditionnels destructifs. *C. R. Soc. Biol.*, 79: 239.

ESTES, W. K. 1943. Discriminative conditioning I. A discriminative property of conditioned anticipation. *J. Exp. Psychol.*, 32: 150.

————. 1948. Discriminative conditioning. II. Effects of a Pavlovian conditioned stimulus upon a subsequently established operant response. *Ibid.*, 38: 173.

————. 1949. A study of the motivating conditions necessary for secondary reinforcement. *Ibid.*, 39: 306.

————. 1950. Toward a statistical theory of learning. *Psychol. Rev.*, 57: 94.

ESTES, W. K., and SKINNER, B. F. 1941. Some quantitative properties of anxiety. *J. Exp. Psychol.*, 29: 390.

ESTES, W K., and STRAUGHAN, J. H. 1954. Analysis of a verbal conditioning situation in terms of statistical learning theory. *J. Exp. Psychol.*, 47: 225.

EYSENCK, H. J. 1947. *Dimensions of Personality*. Routledge & Kegan Paul.

————. 1952. *Scientific Study of Personality*. Routledge & Kegan Paul.

————. 1955. The inheritance of extraversion-introversion. *Acta Psychol.*, 12: 95.

————. 1957. *The Dynamics of Anxiety and Hysteria*. Routledge & Kegan Paul.

————. 1960. *Behavior Therapy and the Neuroses*. Pergamon.

————. 1963. Behavior therapy, extinction and relapse in neuroses. *Brit. J. Psychiat.*, 109: 12.

FARBER, I. E., and SPENCE, K. W. 1953. Complex learning and conditioning as a function of anxiety. *J. Exp. Psychol.*, 45: 120.

FEILBACH, W. 1914. Zur Untersuchung der Assoziationen bei Dementia Paralytica. *Klin. Psych. Nerv. Krank*, 9: 97.

FERSTER, C. B. 1961. Positive reinforcement and behavioral deficits of autistic children. *Child Developm.*, 32: 437.

FIGAR, S. 1959. Some basic deficiencies of the plethysmographic method and possibilities of avoiding them. *Angiology*, 10: 120.

FINAN, J. L. 1940. Quantitative studies in motivation. I. Strength of conditioning in rats under varying degrees of hunger. *J. Comp. Psychol.*, 29: 119.

FINCH, G. 1936. "Hunger" as a factor determining the magnitude of conditioned and unconditioned salivary responses. *Amer. J. Psychol.*, 116: 49.

———. 1938. Hunger as a determinant of conditional and unconditional salivary response magnitude. *Ibid.*, 123: 379.

———. 1938. Pilocarpine conditioning. *Ibid.*, 124: 679.

———. 1938. Salivary conditioning in atropinized dogs. *Ibid.*, p. 136.

FINCH, G., and CULLER, E. 1934. Higher order conditioning with constant motivation. *Amer. J. Psychol.*, 46: 596.

———. 1935. Relation of forgetting to experimental extinction. *Ibid.*, 47: 656.

FINESINGER, J. E., SUTHERLAND, G. F., and McGUIRE, F. F. 1942. The positive conditional salivary reflex in psychoneurotic patients. *Amer. J. Psychiat.*, 99: 61.

FINK, J. B., and PATTON, R. M. 1953. Decrement of a learned drinking response accompanying changes in several stimulus characteristics. *J. Comp. Physiol. Psychol.*, 46: 23.

FISH, F. J. 1958. Leonhard's classification of schizophrenia *J. Ment. Sci.*, 104: 943.

FISHER, V. E. 1932. Hypnotic suggestion and the conditioned reflex. *J. Exp. Psychol.*, 15: 212.

FISHGOLD, H., and GASTAUT, H. (eds.). 1957. Conditionnement et réactivité en électroencéphalographie. *Electroencephalog. Clin. Neurophysiol.*, Suppl. 6.

FITZWATER, M. E., and REISMAN, M. N. 1952. Comparison of forward, simultaneous, backward and pseudo-conditioning. *J. Exp. Psychol.*, 44: 211.

FITZWATER, M. E., and THRUSH, R. S. 1956. Acquisition of a conditioned response as a function of forward temporal contiguity. *J. Exp. Psychol.*, 51: 59.

FLECK, S. 1953. The cardiac component of orienting behavior: response to stimuli of varying intensity. *J. Gen. Psychol.*, 48: 163.

———. 1953. Vigilance (orienting behavior), conditional reactions, and adjustment patterns in schizophrenic and compulsive patients. *Ann. N.Y. Acad. Sci.*, 56: 342.

FLECK, S., and GANTT, W. H. 1951. Conditional responses in patients receiving electric shock treatment. *Amer. J. Psychiat.*, 108: 280.

———. 1949. Fractional conditioning of behavior based on electrically induced convulsions. *Fed. Proc.*, 8: 47.

FRANKS, C. M. 1956. Conditioning and personality: a study of normal and neurotic subjects. *J. Abnorm. Soc. Psychol.*, 52: 143.

———. 1957. Effect of food, drink and tobacco deprivation on the conditioning of the eyeblink response. *J. Exp. Psychol.*, 53: 117.

———. 1957. Personality factors and the rate of conditioning. *J. Psychol.*, 48: 119.

FRANKS, C. M., TROUTON, D. S., and LAVERTY, S. G. 1958. The inhibition of a conditional response following arecoline administration in man. *J. Clin. Exp. Psychopathol.*, 19: 226.

FRANKS, C. M., and WITHERS, W. C. R. 1955. Photoelectric recording of eyelid movements. *Amer. J. Psychol.*, 68: 467.

FREEMAN, G. L. 1930. The galvanic phenomenon and conditioned responses. *J. Gen. Psychol.*, 3: 529.

FREEMAN, W., and WATTS, J. W. 1946. Physiological psychology. *Amer. Rev. Physiol.*, 6: 517.

FREIEROV, O. E. 1954. Problems of the dynamics of oligophrenia. (Rus.) *Z. Nevropat. Psikhiat. (Korsakoff)*, 54: 143.

———. 1956. Pathophysiological mechanisms of oligophrenia. (Rus.) *Z. Vyss. Nerv. Dejat. Pavlova*, 6: 812.

FRENCH, J. D., HERNANDEZ-PEON, R., and LIVINGSTON, R. B. 1955. Projections from cortex to cephalic brain stem (reticular formation) in monkey. *J. Neurophysiol.*, 18: 74.

FROLOV, Y. P. 1937. *Pavlov and His School.* Kegan Paul.

FULTON, J. F. 1949. *Physiology of the Nervous System.* 3d ed. Oxford University Press.

GAGNE, R. M. 1941. The effect of spacing trials on the acquisition and extinction of a conditioned operant response. *J. Exp. Psychol.*, 29: 201.

GAKKEL, L. B., and ZININA, N. V. 1953. Changes of higher nerve function in people over 60 years of age. *Fiziol. Zh. SSSR*, 39: 533.

GALAMBOS, R., SHEATZ, G., and VERNIER, V. G. 1956. Electrophysiological correlates of a conditioned response in cats. *Science*, 123: 376.

GANTT, W. H. 1927. Recent work of Pavlov and his pupils. *Arch. Neurol. Psychiat.*, 17: 514.

———. 1935. Effect of alcohol on cortical and subcortical activity measured by conditioned reflex method. *Bull. Johns Hopkins Hosp.*, 56: 61.

———. 1936. An experimental approach to psychiatry. *Amer. J. Psychiat.*, 92: 1007.

———. 1937. Essential anatomical structures of the reflex arc for establishment of conditioned reflexes. *Amer. J. Physiol.*, 119: 313.

———. 1938. Adaptation to a conditioned reflex pattern. *Fiziol. Zh. SSSR*, 24: 423.

———. 1938. Extension of a conflict based on food to other physiological systems and its reciprocal relations with sexual functions. *Amer. J. Physiol.*, 123: 73.

———. 1938. A method of testing cortical adaptability as measured by a simple conditioned reflex test in certain psychogenic contrasted with organic diseases. *South. Med. Jour.*, 31: 1219.

————. 1938. A method of testing cortical function and sensitivity of the skin. *Arch. Neurol. Psychiat.*, 40: 79.

————. 1940. Effect of alcohol on sexual reflexes in dogs. *Amer. J. Physiol.*, 129: 360.

————. 1940. Relation of unconditioned and conditioned reflex: effect of prolongation of the work period from the usual one hour to a period of ten to twenty hours. *J. Gen. Psychol.*, 23: 377.

————. 1942. Cardiac conditioned reflexes to painful stimuli. *Fed. Proc.*, 1: 28.

————. 1942. The origin and development of nervous disturbances experimentally produced. *Amer. J. Psychiat.*, 98: 475.

————. 1946. Cardiac conditional responses to time. *Trans. Amer. Neurol. Assoc.*, 72: 166.

————. 1948. A physiological basis for nervous dysfunction. *Bull. Johns Hopkins Hosp.*, 8: 416.

————. 1948. Physiological psychology. *Ann. Rev. Physiol.*, 10: 453.

————. 1952. Effect of alcohol on the sexual reflexes of normal and neurotic male dogs. *Psychosom. Med.*, 14: 174.

————. 1953. Principles of nervous breakdown—schizokinesis and autokinesis. *Ann. N.Y. Acad. Sci.*, 56: 143.

————. 1957. Normal and abnormal adaptations—homeostasis, schizokinesis and autokinesis. *Dis. Nerv. Syst.*, 18: 30.

————. 1957. Pavlovian principles and psychiatry. *Prog. Psychother.*, 2: 140.

————. 1957. Pharmacological agents in study of higher nervous activity. *Dis. Nerv. Syst.*, 18: 339.

————. (ed.). 1957. *Physiological Basis of Psychiatry*. Charles C Thomas.

————. 1959. Application of the conditioned reflex method to preventive psychiatry. *Dis. Nerv. Syst.*, 20: 30.

GANTT, W. H., and DYKMAN, R. A. 1952. Experimental psychogenic tachycardia. *Amer. J. Physiol.*, 171: 725.

GANTT, W. H., and FLEISCHMANN, W. 1948. Effect of thyroid therapy on the conditional reflex function in hypothyroidism. *Amer. J. Psychiat.*, 104: 673.

GANTT, W. H., and FREILE, M. 1944. Effect of adrenalin and acetylcholine on excitation, inhibition and neuroses. *Trans. Amer. Neurol. Assoc.* 69: 180.

GANTT, W. H., and HOFFMANN, W. C. 1940. Conditioned cardiorespiratory changes accompanying conditioned food reflexes. *Amer. J. Physiol.*, 129: 360.

GANTT, W. H., and LOUCKS, R. B. 1938. Posterior nerve function as tested by conditioned reflex method. *Amer. J. Physiol.*, 123: 74.

GANTT, W. H., and MUNCIE, W. 1941. Rhythmic variations of muscular activity in normal and neurotic dogs correlated with secretion and with conditioned reflexes. *Amer. J. Physiol.*, 133: 287.

————. 1942. Analysis of the mental defect in chronic Korsakov's psychosis by means of the conditional reflex method. *Bull. Johns
Hopkins Hosp.*, 70: 467.

GANTT, W. H., and TRAUGOTT, U. 1949. Retention of cardiac, salivary and
motor conditional reflexes. *Amer. J. Psysiol.*, 159: 569.

GARLANOVA, T. T., *et al.* 1958. Clinical-physiological data on some types
of internal inhibition in neurasthenic and hysteric patients.
(Rus.) *Tr. Inst. Fiziol. Im. I.P. Pavlov*, 7: 72.

GARVEY, C. R. 1933. A study of conditioned respiratory changes. *J. Exp.
Psychol.*, 16: 471.

GASTAUT, H. 1957. Etat actuel des connaissances sur l'électroencéphalographie du conditionnement. *Electroencephalog. Clin. Neurophysiol.*, Suppl., 6: 133.

————. 1958. Données actuelles sur les mechanismes physiologiques cen-
traux de l'emotion. Rapport du 15eme Congrès International
de Psychologie, 1957. *Bruxelles Psychol. Franç.*, 3: 1.

————. 1958. The role of the reticular formation in establishing conditioned reactions. In *Reticular Formation of the Brain*. Little,
Brown.

————. 1958. Some aspects of the neurophysiological basis of conditioned
reflexes and behavior. In *Neurophysiological Bases of Behavior*.
Churchill.

GASTAUT, H., *et al.* 1956. A topographical study of conditioned electroencephalographic reactions which occur independently, simultaneously or successively in different cortical regions in man.
Electroencephalog. Clin. Neurophysiol., 8: 728.

GASTAUT, H., *et al.* 1957. Electroencephalographic characteristics of the
formation of conditioned reflexes in man. (Rus.) *Fiziol. Zh.
SSSR*, 7: 25.

GASTAUT, H., *et al.* 1957. Etude topographique des réactions électroencéphalographiques conditionnées chez l'homme. *Electroencephalog. Clin. Neurophysiol.*, 9: 1.

GASTAUT, H., *et al.* 1957. Neurophysiological interpretation of conditioned
electroencephalographic reactions. (Rus.) *Fiziol. Zh. SSSR*,
7: 185.

GASTAUT, H., *et al.* 1957. Signification des réactions électroencéphalographiques conditionnées chez l'homme. (Rus.) *Fiziol. Zh.
SSSR*, 7: 185.

GAVLICHEK, V. 1958. Electroencephalographic characteristics of the defensive conditioned reflex. (Rus.) *Fiziol. Zh. SSSR*, 46: 4.

GELLER, I., SIDMAN, M., and BRADY, J. V. 1955. The effect of electro-
convulsive shock on a conditioned emotional response: a control for acquisition recency. *J. Comp. Physiol. Psychol.*, 48:
130.

GELLHORN, E. 1946. Is restoration of inhibited conditioned reactions by insulin coma specific for Pavlovian inhibitions? *Arch. Neurol. Psychiat.*, 56: 216.

GERALL, A. A., SAMPSON, P. B., and BOSLOV, G. L. 1957. Classical conditioning of human pupillary dilation. *J. Exp. Psychol.*, 54: 467.

GERSUNI, G. V., and KOROTKIN, I. I. 1947. Subliminal conditioned reflexes to sound stimuli. (Rus.) *Dokl. Akad. Nauk SSSR*, 59: 417.

GESELL, A. 1938. The conditioned reflex and the psychiatry of infancy. *Amer. J. Orthopsychiat.*, 8: 19.

GESELL, A., *et al.* 1940. *The First Five Years of Life.* Harper.

GIBSON, J. J. 1936. A note on conditioning of voluntary reactions. *J. Exp. Psychol.*, 19: 397.

GIRDEN, E. 1938. Conditioning and problem-solving behavior. *Amer. J. Psychol.*, 51: 677.

———. 1940. Cerebral mechanisms in conditioning under curare. *Ibid.*, 53: 397.

———. 1942. The dissociation of blood pressure conditioned responses under erythroidine. *J. Exp. Psychol.*, 31: 219.

———. 1942. The dissociation of pupillary conditioned reflexes under erythroidine and curare. *Ibid.*, p. 322.

———. 1942. Generalized conditioned responses under curare and erythroidine. *Ibid.*, p. 105.

GIRDEN, E., and CULLER, E. 1937. Conditioned responses in curarized striate muscle in dogs. *J. Comp. Psychol.*, 23: 261.

GIRDEN, E., METTLER, F. A., FINCH, G., and CULLER, E. 1936. Conditioned responses in a decorticate dog to acoustic, thermal, and tactile stimulation. *J. Comp. Psychol.*, 21: 367.

GLASER, GILBERT H. (ed.). 1963. *EEG and Behavior.* Basic Books.

GLEIDMAN, L. H., GANTT, W. H., and TEITELBAUM, H. A. 1957. Some implications of conditional reflex studies for placebo research. *Amer. J. Psychiat.*, 113: 1103.

GLOOR, P. 1955. Electrophysiological studies on the connections of the amygdaloid nucleus in the cat. Part I: The neuronal organization of the amygdaloid projection system. Part II: The electrophysiological properties of the amygdaloid projection system. *Electroencephalog. Clin. Neurophysiol.*, 7: 223.

GOLDRING, S., and O'LEARY, J. L. 1957. Cortical D.C. changes incident to midline thalamic stimulation. *Electroencephalog. Clin. Neurophysiol.*, 9: 577.

GOODRICH, K. P., ROSS, L. E., and WAGNER, A. R. 1957. Performance in eyelid conditioning following interpolated presentations of the US. *J. Exp. Psychol.*, 53: 214.

GOODWIN, J., LONG, L., and WELCH, L. 1945. Generalization in memory. *J. Exp. Psychol.*, 35: 71.

GRAHAM, C. H., and GAGNE, R. M. 1940. The acquisition, extinction and spontaneous recovery of a conditioned operant response. *J. Exp. Psychol.*, 26: 251.

GRAHAM, FRANCES K. 1943. Conditioned inhibition and conditioned excitation in transfer of discrimination. *J. Exp. Psychol.*, 33: 351.

GRANT, D. A. 1939. The influence of attitude on the conditioned eyelid response. *J. Exp. Psychol.*, 25: 333.

————. 1943. The pseudo-conditioned eyelid response. *Ibid.*, 32: 139.

————. 1943. Sensitization and association in eyelid conditioning. *Ibid.*, p. 201.

GRANT, D. A., and ADAMS, J. K. 1944. "Alpha" conditioning in the eyelid. *J. Exp. Psychol.*, 34: 136.

GRANT, D. A., and DITTMER, D. G. 1940. An experimental investigation of Pavlov's cortical irradiation hypothesis. *J. Exp. Psychol.*, 26: 299.

————. 1940. A tactile generalization gradient for pseudo-conditioned response. *Ibid.*, p. 404.

GRANT, D. A., HAKE, H. W., and HORNSETH, J. P. 1951. Acquisition and extinction of a verbal conditioned response with differing percentages of reinforcement. *J. Exp. Psychol.*, 42: 1.

GRANT, D. A., HORNSETH, J. P., and HAKE, H. W. 1950. The influence of the inter-trial interval of the Humphrey's "random reinforcement" effect during the extinction of a verbal response. *J. Exp. Psychol.*, 40: 609.

GRANT, D. A., and NORRIS, EUGENIA B. 1947. Eyelid conditioning as influenced by the presence of sensitized "Beta"-responses. *J. Exp. Psychol.*, 37: 423.

GRANT, D. A., RIOPELLE, A. J., and HAKE, H. W. 1950. Resistance to extinction and the pattern of reinforcement. I. Alternation of reinforcement and the conditioned eyelid response. *J. Exp. Psychol.*, 40: 53.

GRANT, D. A., and SCHILLER, J. J. 1953. Generalization of the conditioned galvanic skin response to visual stimuli. *J. Exp. Psychol.*, 46: 309.

GRANT, D. A., and SCHIPPER, L. M. 1952. The acquisition and extinction of conditioned eyelid responses as a function of the percentage of fixed-ratio random reinforcement. *J. Exp. Psychol.*, 43: 313.

GRANT, D. A., SCHIPPER, L. M., and ROSS, B. M. 1952. Effect of inter-trial interval during acquisition on extinction of the conditioned eyelid response following partial reinforcement. *J. Exp. Psychol.*, 44: 203.

GRANT, D. A., and SCHNEIDER, D. E. 1949. Intensity of the conditioned stimulus and strength of conditioning: the conditioned galvanic skin response to an auditory stimulus. *J. Exp. Psychol.*, 39: 35.

GRASTYAN, E., *et al.* 1958. Beitrage zur Physiologie des Hippocampus. *Physiol. Bohemosl.*, 7: 9.

GRASTYÁN, E., LISSÁK, K., and KÉKESI, F. 1956. Facilitation and inhibition of conditioned alimentary and defensive reflexes by stimulation of the hypothalamus and reticular formation. *Acta Physiol. Hung.*, 9: 133.

GRASTYÁN, E., LISSÁK, K., and SZABO, J. 1954. Funktionelle Zusammenhange Zwischen den Hemmungs—und Aktivierungssystemen des Grosshirns. *Acta Physiol. Hung.*, Suppl., 6: 29.

———. 1955. Cortical electrical manifestations of diencephalic inhibition. *Ibid.*, 7: 187.

GREEN, J. D., and ARDUINI, A. 1954. Hioppocampal electrical activity in arousal. *J. Neurophysiol.*, 17: 14.

GREGORY, IAN. 1961. *Psychiatry—Biological and Social.* Saunders.

GUTHRIE, E. R. 1930. Conditioning as a principle of learning. *Psychol. Rev.*, 37: 412.

———. 1933. Association as a function of time interval. *Ibid.*, 40: 355.

———. 1934. Pavlov's theory of conditioning. *Ibid.*, 41: 199.

———. 1935. *The Psychology of Learning.* Harper.

———. 1938. *The Psychology of Human Conflict.* Harper.

———. 1952. *The Psychology of Learning.* Rev. ed. Harper.

HALL, J. F. 1951. Studies in secondary reinforcement. I. Secondary reinforcement as a function of the frequency of primary reinforcement. *J. Comp. Physiol. Psychol.*, 44: 246.

———. 1951. Studies in secondary reinforcement. II. Secondary reinforcement as a function of the strength of drive during primary reinforcement. *Ibid.*, p. 462.

HAMEL, I. 1919. A study and analysis of the conditioned reflex. *Psychol. Monogr.*, 27: 118.

HARLOW, H. F. 1939. Forward conditioning, backward conditioning and pseudo-conditioning in the goldfish. *J. Genet. Psychol.*, 55: 49.

———. 1940. The effects of incomplete curare paralysis upon formation and elicitation of conditioned responses in cats. *Ibid.*, 56: 273.

———. 1949. The formation of learning sets. *Psychol. Rev.*, 56: 51.

———. 1950. Analysis of discrimination learning by monkeys. *J. Exp. Psychol.*, 40: 26.

———. 1952. Learning. *Ann. Rev. Psychol.*, 3: 29.

HARLOW, H. F., and SETTLAGE, P. H. 1939. The effect of curarization of the fore part of the body upon the retention of conditioned responses in cats. *J. Comp. Psychol.*, 27: 45.

HARLOW, H. F., and TOLTZIEN, F. 1940. Formation of pseudo-conditioned responses in the cat. *J. Gen. Psychol.*, 23: 367.

HARRIS, J. D. 1941. Forward conditioning, backward conditioning, and pseudo-conditioning, and adaptation to the conditioned stimulus. *J. Exp. Psychol.*, 28: 491.

HARZSTEIN, N. G. 1951. Phasic states in the cerebral cortex of patients suffering from reactive depressions. (Rus.) *Z. Vyss. Nerv. Dejat. Pavlova*, 1: 280.

————. 1952. Disturbances of interaction between the first and second signaling systems in reactive depressions. *Ibid.*, 2: 868.

————. 1955. Treatment of reactive depression with prolonged sleep. (Rus.) *Tr. Inst. Vyss. Nerv. Dejat. Ser. Patofiziol.*, 1: 314.

HARZSTEIN, N. G., and TRAUGOTT, N. N. 1940. Changes of the cortical functions of schizophrenics in prolonged narcosis. (Rus.) *Tr. Psikhiat. Klin. I.P. Pavlov*, 2: 227.

HEARST, E., BEER, B., SHEATZ, G., and GALAMBOS, R. 1960. Some electro-physiological correlates of conditioning in the monkey. *Electroencephalog. Clin. Neurophysiol.*, 137: 12.

HEBB, D. O. 1946. Emotion in man and animal: an analysis of the intuitive process of recognition. *Psychol. Rev.*, 53: 88.

————. 1947. Spontaneous neurosis in chimpanzees: theoretical relations with clinical and experimental phenomena. *Psychosom. Med.*, 9: 3.

————. 1949. *The Organization of Behavior.* Wiley.

HERNANDEZ-PEON, R. 1960. Neurophysiological correlates of habituation and other manifestations of plastic inhibition. *Electroencephalog. Clin. Neurophysiol.*, Suppl., 13: 101.

HERNANDEZ-PEON, R., *et al.* 1956. Functional role of brain stem reticular system in salivary conditioned response. *Fed. Proc.*, 15: 91.

HERNANDEZ-PEON, R. *et al.* 1958. Habituation in the visual pathway. *Acta Neurol. Latinoamer.*, 4: 121.

HERNANDEZ-PEON, R., JOUVET, M., and SCHERRER, H. 1957. Auditory potentials at cochlear nucleus during acoustic habituation. *Acta Neurol. Latinoamer.*, 3: 144.

HILDEN, A. H. 1937. An action-current study of the conditioned hand withdrawal. *Psychol. Monogr.*, 49: 173.

HILGARD, E. R. 1931. Conditioned eyelid reactions to a light stimulus based on the reflex wink to sound. *Psychol. Monogr.*, 41: 184.

————. 1933. Modification of reflexes and conditioned reactions. *J. Gen. Psychol.*, 9: 210.

————. 1933. Reinforcement and inhibition of eyelid reflexes. *Ibid.*, 8: 85.

————. 1936. The latency of conditioned eyelid reactions: a reply to Dr. Cason. *J. Exp. Psychol.*, 17: 899.

————. 1936. The nature of the conditioned response. I. The case for and against stimulus substitution. *Psychol. Rev.*, 43: 366.

————. 1936. The nature of the conditioned response. II. Alternatives to stimulus-substitution. *Ibid.*, p. 547.

————. 1937. The relationship between the conditioned response and conventional experiments. *Psychol. Bull.*, 34: 61.

————. 1938. An algebraic analysis of conditioned discrimination in man. *Psychol. Rev.*, 45: 472.

————. 1938. A summary and evaluation of alternative procedures for the construction of Vincent Curves. *Psychol. Bull.*, 35: 282.

————. 1956. *Theories of Learning.* 2d ed. Appleton-Century-Crofts.

HILGARD, E. R., and ALLEN, M. K. 1938. An attempt to condition finger reaction based on motor point stimulation. *J. Gen. Psychol.,* 18: 203.

HILGARD, E. R., and BIEL, W. C. 1937. Reflex sensitization and conditioning of eyelid responses at intervals near simultaneity. *J. Gen. Psychol.,* 16: 223.

HILGARD, E. R., and CAMPBELL, A. A. 1936. The course of acquisition and retention of conditioned eyelid responses in man. *J. Exp. Psychol.,* 19: 227.

HILGARD, E. R., CAMPBELL, A. A., and SEARS, W. N. 1937. Conditioned discrimination: the development of discrimination with and without verbal report. *Amer. J. Psychol.,* 49: 564.

————. 1938. Conditioned discrimination: the effect of knowledge of stimulus-relationship. *Ibid.,* 51: 498.

HILGARD, E. R., and HUMPHREYS, L. G. 1938. The retention of conditioned discrimination in man. *J. Gen. Psychol.,* 19: 111.

HILGARD, E. R., and MARQUIS, D. G. 1935. Acquisition, extinction, and retention of conditioned lid responses to light in dogs. *J. Comp. Psychol.,* 19: 29.

————. 1936. Conditioned eyelid responses in monkeys, with a comparison of dog, monkey and man. *Psychol. Monogr.,* 47: 186.

————. 1940. *Conditioning and Learning.* Appleton-Century-Crofts.

HILGARD, E. R., MILLER, J., and OHLSON, J. A. 1933. Three attempts to secure pupillary conditioning to auditory stimuli near the absolute threshold. *J. Exp. Psychol.,* 16: 283.

HOVLAND, C. I. 1937. The generalization of conditioned responses. I. The sensory generalization of conditioned responses with varying frequencies of tone. *J. Gen. Psychol.,* 17: 125.

————. 1937. The generalization of conditioned responses. II. The sensory generalization of conditioned responses with varying intensities of tone. *J. Genet. Psychol.,* 51: 279.

————. 1937. The generalization of conditioned responses. III. Extinction, spontaneous recovery, and disinhibition of conditioned and generalized responses. *J. Exp. Psychol.,* 21: 47.

————. 1937. The generalization of conditioned responses. IV. The effects of varying amounts of reinforcement upon the degrees of generalization of conditioned responses. *Ibid.,* p. 261.

HOVLAND, C. I., and RIESAN, A. H. 1940. Magnitude of galvanic and vasomotor response as a function of stimulus intensity. *J. Gen. Psychol.* 23: 103.

HUDGINS, C. V. 1933. Conditioning and the voluntary control of the pupillary light reflex. *J. Gen. Psychol.,* 8: 3.

————. 1935. Steckle and Renshaw on the conditioned iridic reflex: a discussion. *Ibid.,* 12: 208.

HUGHES, B., and SCHLOSBERG, H. 1939. Conditioning in the white rat. IV. The conditioned lid reflex. *J. Exp. Psychol.*, 23: 641.

HULL, C. L. 1929. A functional interpretation of the conditioned reflex. *Psychol. Rev.*, 36: 498.

————. 1930. Simple trial-and-error learning: a study in psychological theory. *Ibid.*, 37: 241.

————. 1933. Differential habituation to internal stimuli in the albino rat. *J. Comp. Psychol.*, 16: 255.

————. 1935. The mechanism of the assembly of behavior segments in novel combinations suitable for problem solution. *Ibid.*, p. 219.

————. 1935. The conflicting psychologies of learning—a way out. *Psychol. Rev.*, 42: 491.

————. 1935. Thorndike's fundamentals of learning. *Psychol. Bull.*, 32: 807.

————. 1937. Mind mechanism and adaptive behavior. *Psychol. Rev.*, 44: 1.

————. 1939. The problem of stimulus—equivalence in behavior theory. *Ibid.*, 46: 9.

————. 1940. Explorations in the patterning of stimuli conditioned to the G.S.R. *J. Exp. Psychol.*, 27: 95.

————. 1943. *Principles of Behavior*. Appleton-Century-Crofts.

————. 1947. The problem of primary stimulus generalization. *Psychol. Rev.*, 54: 120.

————. 1951. *Essentials of Behavior*. Yale Univ. Press.

————. 1952. *A Behavior System*. Yale Univ. Press.

HUMPHREY, G. 1920. The conditioned reflex and the Freudian wish. *J. Abnorm. Soc. Psychol.*, 14: 389.

————. 1921. Education and Freudianism: the Freudian mechanism and the conditioned reflex. *Ibid.*, 15: 350.

————. 1928. The conditioned reflex and the laws of learning. *J. Educ. Psychol.*, 19: 424.

HUMPHREYS, L. G. 1939. Acquisition and extinction of verbal expectations in a situation analogous to conditioning. *J. Exp. Psychol.*, 25: 294.

————. 1939. Generalization as a function of method of reinforcement *Ibid.*, p. 361.

HUMPHREYS, L. G., MILLER, J., and ELLSON, D. G. 1940. The effect of inter-trial interval on the acquisition, extinction, and recovery of verbal expectation. *J. Exp. Psychol.*, 27: 195.

HUNT, E. L. 1949. Establishment of conditioned responses in chick embryos. *J. Comp. Physiol. Psychol.*, 42: 107.

HUNT, H. F. 1956. Some effects of drugs on classical (type S) conditioning. *Ann. N.Y. Acad. Sci.*, 65: 258.

————. 1957. Some effects of meprobamate on conditional fear and emotional behavior. *Ibid.*, 67: 712.

HUNT, H. F., JERNBERG, P., and LAWLOR, W. G. 1953. The effect of electro-convulsive shock on a conditional emotional response: the effect of electro-convulsive shock under ether anaesthesia. *J. Comp. Physiol. Psychol.*, 46: 64.

HUNT, H. F., JERNBERG, P., and OTIS, L. S. 1953. The effect of carbon disulphide convulsions on a conditioned emotional response. *J. Comp. Physiol. Psychol.*, 46: 465.

HUNTER, W. S. 1928. *Human Behavior.* Univ. Chicago Press.

———. 1935. A curve of experimental extinction in the white rat. *Science,* 82: 374.

———. 1935. Conditioning and extinction in the rat. *Brit. J. Psychol.*, 26: 135.

———. 1935. Conditioning and maze learning in the rat. *J. Comp. Psychol.*, 19: 417.

———. 1936. Learning curves for conditioning and maze learning. *J. Exp. Psychol.*, 19: 156.

———. 1937. Muscle potentials and conditioning in the rat. *Ibid.*, 21: 611.

———. 1938. An experiment on the disinhibition of voluntary responses. *Ibid.*, 22: 419.

IRWIN, O. C. 1939. Toward a theory of conditioning. *Psychol. Rev.*, 46: 425.

ISSERLIN, M. 1907. Psychologische Untersuchungen an Manisch-depressiven. *Mschr. Psychiat. Neurol.*, 22: 302.

IVANOV-SMOLENSKY, A. G. 1922. The biogenesis of speech reflexes and the fundamental methodological principles of investigation. (Rus.) *Psikhiat. Nevropatol. Eksp. Psikol.*, 2: 231.

———. 1925. Experimentelle Untersuchungen über sprachliche und mimische Reflexe in der manischen Phase der Cyklophrenie. *Z. Ges. Neurol. Psychiat.*, 98: 680.

———. 1925. Uber die Bedingten Reflexe in der Depressiven Phase des Manische Depressiven Irreseins. *Mschr. Psychiat. Neurol.*, 58: 376.

———. 1927. Etudes expérimentales sur les enfants et les aliénés selon la méthode des réflexes conditionnels. *Ann. Méd. Psychol.*, 85: 140.

———. 1927. On the methods of examining the conditional food reflexes in children and in mental disorders. *Brain,* 50: 138.

———. 1927. Neurotic behavior and teaching of conditional reflexes. *Amer. J. Psychiat.*, 84: 483.

———. 1928. Pathology of conditional reflexes and so-called psychogenic depression. *J. Nerv. Ment. Dis.*, 67: 346.

———. 1928. Uber Pathophysiologische Grundmechanismen der Psychoneurosen. *Schweiz. Arch. Neurol. Psychiat.*, 22: 13.

———. 1934. An attempt at pathophysiological study of mutism in schizophrenia. (Rus.) *Ark Biol. Nauk,* Ser. B., 36: 107.

————. 1935. Concerning different forms and neuro-dynamics of catatonic stupor. *Ibid.*, p. 85.

————. 1951. Concerning the study of the joint activity of the first and second signalling system. (Rus.) *Z. Vyss. Nerv. Dejat. Pavlova*, 1: 55.

————. 1953. Investigations into the interactions of the first and second signalling systems. *Ibid.*, 3: 481.

————. 1954. *Essays on the Patho-Physiology of the Higher Nervous Activity: According to I.P. Pavlov and His School.* Foreign Languages Publishing House.

————. 1956. Some new data from the study of nervous mechanisms in the interaction of the cortical signalling systems. (Rus.) *Tr. Inst. Vyss. Nerv. Dejat. Ser. Patofiziol.*, 2: 315.

IWAMA, K. 1950. Delayed conditioned reflex in man and brain waves. *Tohoku J. Exp. Med.*, 52: 53.

IWAMA, K., and ABE, M. 1952. Electroencephalographic study of conditioned salivary reflexes in human subjects. *Tohoku J. Exp. Med.*, 56: 345.

————. 1953. Conditioned galvanic skin reflex and electroencephalogram. *Ibid.*, 59: 327.

JACOBSEN, E. 1959. The comparative pharmacology of some psychotropic drugs. *Bull. World Health Organ.*, 21: 411.

JACOBSEN, E., and SONNE, E. 1956. The effect of benactyzine on the conditioned responses in the rat. *Acta Pharmacol. Toxicol.*, 12: 310.

JASPER, H. 1949. Diffuse projection systems: the integrative action of the thalamic reticular system. *Electroencephalog. Clin. Neurophysiol.*, 1: 405.

JASPER, H., and AJMONE-MARSAN, C. 1952. Thalamo-cortical integrating mechanisms. *Assoc. Res. Nerv. Ment. Dis. Proc.*, 30: 493.

JASPER, H., AJMONE-MARSAN, C. A., and STOLL, J. 1952. Symposium on brain and mind; corticofugal projections to brain stem. *Arch. Neurol. Psychiat.*, 67: 155.

JASPER, H., NAQUET, R., and KING, E. E. 1955. Thalamo-cortical recruiting responses in sensory receiving areas in cat. *Electroencephalog. Clin. Neurophysiol.*, 7: 99.

JASPER, H., and SHAGASS, C. 1941. Conditioning the occipital alpha rhythm in man. *J. Exp. Psychol.*, 28: 373.

————. 1941. Conscious time judgments related to conditioned time intervals and voluntary control of the alpha rhythm. *Ibid.*, p. 503.

JASPER, H., and SMIRNOV, G. D. (eds.). 1960. The Moscow Colloquium on Electroencephalography of the Higher Nervous Activity. *Electroencephalog. Clin. Neurophysiol.*, Suppl. 13.

JASPERS, KARL. 1962. *General Psychopathology.* Manchester Univ. Press.

JONES, H. G. 1956. The application of conditioning and learning techniques to the treatment of a psychiatric patient. *J. Abnorm. Soc. Psychol.*, 52: 414.

JOUVET, M., BENOIT, C., and COURJON, J. 1956. EEG studies of the processes of connection formation between a light stimulus and a sound stimulus in the cat. *Electroencephalog. Clin. Neurophysiol.*, 8: 727.

JOUVET, M., and HERNANDEZ-PEON, R. 1957. Mécanismes neurophysiologues concernant l'habituation, l'attention et le conditonnement. *Electroencephalog. Clin. Neurophysiol.*, Suppl. 6, p. 39.

JUS, A., and JUS, C. 1953. Methodological principles of electroencephalographic investigations concerning the process of internal inhibition; retardation and passage into sleep. *Neurol. Neurochir. Psychiat. Polska,* 6: 595.

―――. 1954. Electroencephalographic analysis of the processes of internal inhibition; retardation and transition into sleep. *Ibid.*, 1: 23.

―――. 1956. Bioelectric researches on the formation and transformation of conditoned motor reflexes in the dynamic stereotype. *Ibid.*, 3: 291.

―――. 1957. The significance of electroencephalographic conditional reactions for pathophysiological investigations in neurology and psychiatry. (Rus.) *Z. Nevropat. Psikhiat. (Korsakoff),* 57: 1363.

JUS, C., and JUS, A. 1954. Electroencephalographic and electromyographic analysis of the mechanism of the motor conditioned reflex with application of the Ivanov-Smolensky method. Report I. *Neurol. Neurochir. Psychiat. Polska,* 3: 253.

KALISH, H. I. 1958. The relationship between discriminability and generalization: a re-evaluation. *J. Exp. Psychol.*, 55: 637.

KALISH, H. I., and GUTTMAN, M. 1957. Stimulus generalization after equal training on two stimuli. *J. Exp. Psychol.*, 53: 139.

KAMIN, L. J. 1956. The effects of termination of the CS and avoidance of the US on avoidance learning. *J. Comp. Physiol. Psychol.*, 49: 420.

KAPPAUF, W. E., and SCHLOSBERG, H. 1937. Conditioned responses in the white rat. III. Conditioning as a function of the length of the period of delay. *J. Genet. Psychol.*, 50: 27.

KATZENELBOGEN, S., LOUCKS, R. B., and GANTT, W. H. 1938. Conditioned responses to peripherally acting drugs (histamine). *Amer. J. Physiol.*, 123: 113.

KAWAMURA, Y., and YOSHII, N. 1951. A study on the experimental neurosis of rats: behavior patterns. *Med. J. Osaka Univ.*, 2: 133.

KELLOGG, W. N. 1947. Is "spinal conditioning" conditioning? Reply to a comment. *J. Exp. Psychol.*, 37: 263.

KELLOGG, W. N., DEESE, J., PRONKO, N. H., and FEINBERG, M. 1947. An attempt to condition the chronic spinal dog. *J. Exp. Psychol.*, 37: 99.

KELLOGG, W. N., PRONKO, N. H., and DEESE, J. 1946. Spinal conditioning in dogs. *Science,* 103: 49.

KELLOGG, W. N., SCOTT, V. B., DAVIS, R. C., and WOLF, I. S. 1940. Is movement necessary for learning? *J. Comp. Psychol.,* 29: 43.

KELLOGG, W. N., and WALKER, E. L. 1938. "Ambiguous conditioning," a phenomenon of bilateral transfer. *J. Comp. Psychol.,* 26: 63.

————. 1938. An analysis of the bilateral transfer of conditioning in dogs, in terms of the frequency, amplitude and latency of the responses. *J. Gen. Psychol.,* 18: 253.

KELLOGG, W. N., and WOLF, I. S. 1939. The nature of the response retained after several varieties of conditioning in the same subjects. *J. Exp. Psychol.,* 24: 366.

KENNARD, M. A. 1953. The electroencephalogram in psychological disorders. *Psychosom. Med.,* 15: 95.

KENT, G. H., and ROSANOFF, A. J. 1910. A study of association in insanity. *Amer. J. Insan.,* 67: 37.

KERBIKOV, O. V., and KRYLOV, D. N. 1953. Studies of ultraparadoxical phases in psychogenic reactions. (Rus.) *Z. Vyss. Nerv. Dejat. Pavlova,* 3: 369.

KESSEN, W. 1953. Response strength and conditioned stimulus intensity. *J. Exp. Psychol.,* 45: 82.

KHALETSKY, A. M. 1956. Problems of infectious psychoses in the contemporary psychiatric literature. (Rus.) *Z. Nevropat. Psikhiat. (Korsakoff),* 56: 395.

KHOMUTOV, A. V. 1957. About the investigation methods of conditional speech reflexes. (Rus.) *Z. Vyss. Nerv. Dejat. Pavlova,* 7: 775.

KIMBLE, G. A. 1947. Conditioning as a function of the time between conditioned and unconditioned stimulus. *J. Exp. Psychol.,* 37: 1.

————. 1949. An experimental test of a two-factor theory of inhibition. *Ibid.,* 39: 15.

KIMBLE, G. A., and DUFORT, R. H. 1956. The associative factor in eyelid conditioning. *J. Exp. Psychol.,* 52: 386.

KIMBLE, G. A., MANN, LUCIE I., and DUFORT, R. H. 1955. Classical and instrumental eyelid conditioning. *J. Exp. Psychol.,* 49: 407.

KLEITMAN, N. 1927. The influence of starvation on the rate of secretion of saliva elicited by pilocarpine, and its bearing on conditioned salivation. *Amer. J. Physiol.,* 82: 686.

————. 1939. *Sleep and Wakefulness.* Univ. Chicago Press.

KLEITMAN, N., and CRISLER, G. 1927. A quantitative study of a salivary conditioned reflex. *Amer. J. Physiol.,* 79: 571.

KLÜVER, H. 1933. *Behavior Mechanisms in Monkeys.* Univ. Chicago Press.

KNOTT, J. R. 1941. Electroencephalography and physiological psychology: evaluation and statement of problem. *Psychol. Bull.,* 38: 944.

KNOTT, J. R., and HENRY, C. E. 1941. The conditioning of the blocking of the alpha rhythm of the human electroencephalogram. *J. Exp. Psychol.*, 28: 134.

KNOTT, J. R., PLATT, E. B., and HADLEY, H. D. 1944. A preliminary neurophysiological investigation of the behavioral concept of stimulus trace. *J. Exp. Psychol.*, 34: 104.

KOCH, E. 1932. Die Irradiation der pressorezeptorischen Kreislauf-reflexe. *Klin. Wschr.*, 2: 225.

KOGAN, A. B. 1956. Action potentials in subcortical ganglia during some reflex performances. *Bull. Exp. Biol. Med.*, 2: 130.

―――. 1958. Electrophysiological indices of excitation and inhibition in the cerebral cortex. *Fiziol. Zh. SSSR*, 44: 810.

KOHLER, W. 1925. *The Mentality of Apes.* Harcourt Brace.

KOK, E. P. 1959. Study of the process of generalization in patients with motor and sensory aphasia. (Rus.) *Z. Vyss. Nerv. Dejat. Pavlova*, 9: 14.

KONORSKI, J. 1948. *Conditioned Reflexes and Neuron Organization.* Cambridge Univ. Press.

KONORSKI, J., and MILLER, S. 1937. On two types of conditioned reflex. *J. Gen. Psychol.*, 16: 264.

―――. 1937. Further remarks on two types of conditioned reflex. *Ibid.*, 17: 405.

KOROTKIN, I. I. 1952. The effect of word stimuli as conditional inhibition in alert and hypnotic states. (Rus.) *Tr. Inst. Fiziol. Im. I.P. Pavlov*, 1: 345.

KOROTKIN, I. I., and PLESHKOVA, T. V. 1958. On the difficulties of elaborating conditional inhibition in patients with phobic neuroses. (Rus.) *Tr. Inst. Fiziol. Im. I.P. Pavlov*, 7: 185.

KOROTKIN, I. I., and SUSLOVA, M. M. 1951. Studies of the higher nervous activity in man in the somnambulic stage of hypnosis. (Rus.) *Z. Vyss. Nerv. Dejat. Pavlova*, 1: 617.

―――. 1955. The physiological mechanism of inhibitory action on stimuli inhibited by hypnotic suggeston. (Rus.) *Dokl. Akad. Nauk SSSR*, 1: 189.

―――. 1957. Investigations of posthypnotic changes in conditional and unconditional reflexes resulting from suggestions made in the first phase of the hypnosis. (Rus.) *Z. Vyss. Nerv. Dejat. Pavlova*, 7: 889.

KOSTANDOV, E. A. 1955. Disturbances of the neurodynamics, and especially the interaction of the signaling systems in the paranoid form of schizophrenia. (Rus.) *Tr. Inst. Vyss. Nerv. Dejat. Ser. Patofiziol.*, 1: 26.

―――. 1958. Disturbances of interaction of the first and second signaling systems in the catatonic form of schizophrenia. (Rus.) *Ibid.*, 5: 101.

KOTLIAREVSKY, L. I. 1935. The formation of pupillary conditioned reflexes and of a differentiation in response to both direct and verbal stimuli. (Rus.) *Ark. Biol. Nauk,* 39: 477.

Kovalev, V. V. 1955. Disturbances of the cortical dynamics in the Korsakoff syndrome. (Rus.) *Z. Nevropat. Psikhiat. (Korsakoff),* 55: 765.

Kozhevnikov, A., and Maruseva, A. M. 1949. EEG studies of the formation of temporary connections to subliminal stimuli in man. (Rus.) *Dokl. Akad. Nauk SSSR,* 5: 560.

Kozlov, Y. G. 1953. Pathophysiological mechanism of the hypochondriacal delusions. (Rus.) *Z. Nevropat. Psikhiat. (Korsakoff),* 53: 935.

———. 1958. The influences of aminazine on the basic processes of the higher nervous activity. (Rus.) *Z. Vyss. Nerv. Dejat. Pavlova,* 8: 904.

Krasnogorski, N. I. 1909. Uber die Bedingungsreflexe in Kindesalter. *Jb. Kinderheilk.,* 69: 1.

———. 1913. Uber die Grundmechanismen der Arbeit der Grosshirnrinde bie Kindern. *Ibid.,* 78: 373.

———. 1925. The conditioned reflexes and children's neuroses. *Amer. J. Dis. Child.,* 30: 753.

———. 1952. The physiology of speech development in children. (Rus.) *Z. Vyss. Nerv. Dejat. Pavlova,* 2: 474.

———. 1956. New data on the physiology of speech activity. *Ibid.,* 6: 513.

Kreindler, A., and Fradis, A. 1957. Studies on the neurodynamics of aphasia. (Rus.) *Z. Nevropat. Psikhiat. (Korsakoff),* 57: 929.

Kreindler, A., *et al.* 1958. Electroclinical features of convulsions induced by stimulation on brain stem. *J. Neurophysiol.,* 20: 430.

Kreindler, A., Ungher, J., and Volanschi, D. 1958. Effects of brainstem lesions on higher nervous activity in dogs. (Roumanian) *Studii si Cercet. Neurol.,* 3: 387.

Kreindler, A., and Zuckermann, E. 1955. Characteristics of convulsive seizures caused by focal stimulation of the brainstem. (Roumanian) *Studii si Cercet. Neurol.,* 1: 178.

Kupalov, P. S. 1933. The effect of a system of rhythmic conditioned reflexes on the formation and duration of a new conditioned reflex. (Rus.) *Publ. Pavlov Fiziol. Inst.,* 5: 383.

———. 1933. Excitation of a conditioned reflex with long and short-duration application of the conditioned stimulus. (Rus.) *Ark. Biol. Nauk,* 33: 679.

———. 1933. Periodic excitability changes of cortical tissue during active and inhibitory reflexes. (Rus.) *Publ. Pavlov Fiziol. Inst.,* 5: 355.

———. 1947. The relation of cortical activity to the secretory activity curves. (Rus.) *Fiziol. Zh. SSSR,* 33: 495.

Kupalov, P. S., and Gantt, W. H. 1927. The relationship between the strength of the conditioned stimulus and the size of the resulting conditioned reflex. *Brain*, 50: 44.

KUPALOV, P. S., LYMAN, R. S., and LUKOV, B. N. 1931. The relationship between the intensity of tone-stimuli and the size of the resulting conditioned reflexes. *Brain*, 54: 85.

KUPALOV, P. S., and SKIPIN, G. B. 1934. The effect of frequency of stimulation and the amount of salivary secretion. (Rus.) *Fiziol. Zh. SSSR*, 17: 1301.

KUTIN, V. P. 1956. The problem of pathophysiological characteristics of chronic states of schizophrenia. (Rus.) *Z. Vyss. Nerv. Dejat. Pavlova*, 6: 251.

LACEY, J. I. 1956. The evaluation of autonomic responses: toward a general solution. *Ann. N.Y. Acad. Sci.*, 67: 123.

LACEY, J. I., and SMITH, R. L. 1954. Conditioning and generalization of unconscious anxiety. *Science*, 120: 1045.

LACEY, J. I., SMITH, R. L., and GREEN, A. 1955. Use of conditioned autonomic responses in the study of anxiety. *Psychosom. Med.*, 17: 208.

LAKOSINA, N. D. 1958. Studies of the psychogalvanic skin reactions in schizophrenic patients. (Rus.) *Z. Nevropat. Psikhiat. (Korsakoff)*, 58: 1477.

LANDIS, C. 1932. Electrical phenomena of the skin (galvanic skin response). *Psychol. Bull.*, 29: 693.

LANDIS, C., and DEWICK, H. 1929. The electrical phenomena of the skin (psychogalvanic reflex). *Psychol. Bull.*, 26: 64.

LANG, J. M., and OLMSTED, J. M. D. 1923. Conditioned reflexes and pathways in the spinal cord. *Amer. J. Physiol.*, 65: 603.

LANGFELDT, G. 1953. Some points regarding symptomatology and diagnosis of schizophrenia. *Acta Psychiat. Scand.*, Suppl., 80: 7.

LARSSON, L. 1956. The relation between the startle reaction and the non-specific EEG response to sudden stimuli with a discussion on the mechanism of arousal. *Electroencephalog. Clin. Neurophysiol.*, 8: 631.

LASHLEY, K. S. 1916. The human salivary reflex and its use in psychology. *Psychol. Rev.*, 23: 446.

———. 1916. Reflex secretion of the human parotid gland. *J. Exp. Psychol.*, 1: 461.

———. 1929. *Brain Mechanisms and Intelligence*. Univ. Chicago Press.

———. 1930. Basic neural mechanisms in behavior. *Psychol. Rev.*, 37: 1.

———. 1938. Conditional reactions in the rat. *J. Psychol.*, 6: 311.

LASHLEY, K. S., and WADE, M. 1946. The Pavlovian theory of generalization. *Psychol. Rev.*, 53: 72.

LAST, S. L., and STROM-OLSEN, R. 1936. Chronaximetric studies in catatonia. *J. Ment. Sci.*, 82: 763.

LEDER, S. 1955. Dynamics of unconditional and conditional vegetative reflexes in the course of catatonia stupor. (Pol.) *Neurol. Neurochir. Psychiat. Polska*, 5: 171.

LEEPER, R. 1944. Dr. Hull's principles of behavior. *J. Genet. Psychol.*, 64: 3.

LEHMANN, H. E. 1958. Tranquilizers and other psychotropic drugs in clinical practice. *Can. Med. Assoc. J.*, 79: 701.

———. 1961. New drugs in psychiatric therapy. *Ibid.*, 85: 1145.

LEONHARD, K. 1949. Einige kombinierte-systematische Schizophrenien. *Allg. Z. Psychiat.*, 124: 409.

———. 1952. Formen und Verläufe der Schizophrenien. *Mschr. Psychiat. Neurol.*, 124: 169.

LEPLEY, W. M. 1932. A theory of serial learning and forgetting based upon conditioned reflex principles. *Psychol. Rev.*, 39: 279.

LEVIN, S. L. 1953. Attempt at physiological analysis of depersonalization phenomena in schizophrenia. (Rus.) *Z. Nevropat. Psikhiat. (Korsakoff)*, 53: 847.

LEWIS, D. J. 1956. Acquisition, extinction and spontaneous recovery as a function of percentage of reinforcement and intertrial intervals. *J. Exp. Psychol.*, 51: 45.

LIBERMAN, A. E., and STRELZOVA, N. Y. 1952. Some characteristics of the pupillary component of the orienting reflex. (Rus.) *Z. Vyss. Nerv. Dejat. Pavlova*, 2: 886.

LICHKO, A. E. 1957. Clinical-physiological characteristics of the insulin coma. (Rus.) *Z. Nevropat. Psikhiat. (Korsakoff)*, 57: 1509.

———. 1958. Contributions to the physiological study of amnesia in cases of insulin shocks. (Rus.) *Z. Vyss. Nerv. Dejat. Pavlova*, 8: 793.

LIDDELL, H. S. 1926. A laboratory for the study of conditioned motor reflexes. *Amer. J. Psychol.*, 37: 418.

———. 1936. Pavlov, the psychiatrist of the future. *J. Mt. Sinai Hosp.*, 3: 101.

———. 1938. The experimental neuroses and the problem of mental disorder. *Amer. J. Psychiat.*, 94: 1035.

LIDDELL, H. S., JAMES, W. T., and ANDERSON, O. D. 1934. The comparative physiology of the conditioned motor reflexes: based on experiments with the pig, dog, sheep, goat and rabbit. *Comp. Psychol. Monogr.*, 11: 51.

LIDDELL, H. S., SUTHERLAND, G. F., PARMENTER, R., and BAYNE, T. 1936. A study of the conditioned reflex method for producing experimental neuroses. *Amer. J. Physiol.*, 116: 95.

LIGHT, J. S., and GANTT, W. H. 1936. Essential part of reflex arc for establishment of conditioned reflex: formation of conditioned reflex after exclusion of motor peripheral end. *J. Comp. Psychol.*, 21: 19.

LILLY, J. C. 1957. Learning elicited by electrical stimulation of subcortical regions in the unanesthetized monkey: the "start" and the "stop" patterns of behavior. *Science*, 125: 748.

LINDSLEY, D., BOWDEN, J. W., and MAGOUN, H. W. 1949. Effect upon the EEG of acute injury to the brain stem activating system. *Electroencephalog. Clin. Neurophysiol.*, 1: 475.

LINDSLEY, D., SCHREINER, H., KNOWLES, W. B., and MAGOUN, H. W. 1950. Behavioral and EEG changes following chronic brain stem lesions in the cat. *Electroencephalog. Clin. Neurophysiol.*, 2: 483.

LINDSLEY, O. R. 1956. Operant conditioning methods applied to research in chronic schizophrenia. *Psychiat. Res. Rep.*, 5: 118.

LIPSKAYA, L. A. 1958. Problems of the pathogenesis of reactive psychoses. (Rus.) *Tr. Inst. Fiziol. Im. I.P. Pavlov*, 7: 211.

LISSAK, K., *et al.* 1957. A study of hippocampal function in the waking and sleeping animal with chronically implanted electrodes. *Acta Physiol. Pharmacol. Néerl.*, 6: 451.

LITTMAN, R. A. 1949. Conditioned generalization of the galvanic skin reaction to tones. *J. Exp. Psychol.*, 39: 868.

LITVINOVA, V. E. 1955. Motor chronaxy in schizophrenics in changes of the fundamental dynamics of cortical processes. (Rus.) *Z. Nevropat. Psikhiat. (Korsakoff)*, 55: 259.

LIVANOV, M. N., and POLIAKOV, K. L. 1945. Electrical cortical phenomena in the rabbit during the acquisition of defensive reflex using rhythmical stimuli. (Rus.) *Tr. Akad. Med. Nauk SSSR*, 3: 286.

LOGAN, F. A. 1951. A comparison of avoidance and non-avoidance eyelid conditioning. *J. Exp. Psychol.*, 42: 390.

LOOMIS, A. L., HARVEY, E. N., and HOBART, G. 1936. Electrical potentials of the human brain. *J. Exp. Psychol.*, 19: 249.

———. 1938. Distribution of disturbance patterns in human EEG with special reference to sleep. *J. Neurophysiol.*, 1: 413.

LOUCKS, R. B. 1933. An appraisal of Pavlov's systematization of behavior from the experimental standpoint. *J. Comp. Psychol.*, 15: 1.

———. 1933. An automatic technique for establishing conditioned reflexes. *Amer. J. Psychol.*, 44: 338.

———. 1937. Humeral conditioning in mammals. *J. Psychol.*, 4: 295.

———. 1937. Reflexology and the psychobiological approach. *Psychol. Rev.*, 44: 320.

———. 1938. Studies of neural structures essential for learning. II. The conditioning of salivary and striped muscle responses to faradization of cortical sensory elements and the action of sleep upon such mechanisms. *J. Comp. Psychol.*, 25: 315.

LOUCKS, R. B., and GANTT, W. H. 1938. The conditioning of striped muscle responses based upon faradic stimulation of dorsal roots and dorsal columns of the spinal cord. *J. Comp. Psychol.*, 25: 415.

LOWENBACH, H., and GANTT, W. H. 1940. Conditional vestibular reactions. *J. Neurophysiol.*, 3: 43.

LUKOV, B. N. 1949. The formation of a conditioned reflex following the application of short-duration conditioned stimulus. (Rus.) *Publ. Pavlov Fiziol. Inst.*, 15: 151.

LUMSDAINE, A. A. 1939. Conditioned eyelid responses as mediating generalized conditioned finger reactions. *Psychol. Bull.*, 36: 650.

LUNN, V. 1958. About the influence of electro-shock on the conditional withdrawal-reflex in man. (Dan.) *Nord Psykiat. Medlemsbl.*, Suppl., 1: 249.

McALLISTER, W. R. 1953. Adaptation of the original response to a conditioned stimulus. *Iowa Acad. Sci.*, 60: 534.

————. 1953. The effect on eyelid conditioning of shifting the CS-US interval. *Ibid.*, p. 423.

————. 1953. Eyelid conditioning as a function of the CS-US interval. *J. Exp. Psychol.*, 45: 417.

MacDONALD, ANNETTE. 1946. The effect of adaptation to the unconditioned stimulus upon the formation of conditioned avoidance responses. *J. Exp. Psychol.*, 36: 1.

McGEOCH, J. A., and IRION, A. L. 1952. *The Psychology of Human Learning*. Longmans, Green.

MacLEAN, P. D. 1949. Psychosomatic disease and the "visceral brain." *Psychosom. Med.*, 11: 338.

————. 1954. The limbic system and its hippocampal formation. *J. Neurosurg.*, 11: 29.

MacLEAN, P. D., *et al.* 1955. Hippocampal function: tentative correlations of conditioning, EEG, drug and radioautographic studies. *Yale J. Biol. Med.*, 28: 380.

MacLEAN, P. D., and DELGADO, J. M. R. 1953. Electrical and clinical stimulation of fronto-temporal portion of limbic system in the waking animal. *Electroencephalog. Clin. Neurophysiol.*, 5: 91.

MAGOUN, H. W. 1958. *The Waking Brain*. Charles C Thomas.

MALMO, R. B., *et al.* 1951. Electromyographic studies of muscular tension in psychiatric patients under stress. *J. Clin. Exp. Psychopathol.*, 12: 45.

MALMO, R. B., and SHAGASS, C. 1940. Physiologic studies of reaction to stress in anxiety and early schizophrenia. *Psychosom. Med.*, 11: 9.

MALMO, R. B., SHAGASS, C., and SMITH, A. A. 1951. Responsiveness in chronic schizophrenia. *J. Personality*, 19: 359.

MARINESCO, G. 1937. Contribution à l'étude des troubles sensitifs hystériques et le rôle des réflexes conditionnels dans la physio-pathologie de l'hystérie. *Rev. Neurol.*, 68: 585.

MARINESCO, G., and KREINDLER, A. 1934. *Des Reflexes Conditionnels*. Alcan.

MARINESCO, G., KREINDLER, A., and COPELMAN, L. 1935. Le test de Rorschach et la dynamique de l'écorce cérébrale d'après les lois des réflexes conditionnels de Pavlov. *Ann. Méd. Psychol.*, 93: 614.

MARKUS, O. 1911. Uber associationen bei Dementia praecox. *Arch. Psychiat. Nervenkr.*, 48: 344.

MARQUIS, D. G. 1931. Can conditioned responses be established in the newborn infant? *J. Genet Psychol.*, 39: 479.

MARQUIS, D. G., and HILGARD, E. R. 1936. Conditioned lid responses to light in dogs after removal of the visual cortex. *J. Comp. Psychol.*, 22: 157.

MARQUIS, D. G., and PORTER, J. M., JR. 1939. Differential characteristics of conditioned eyelid responses established by reflex and voluntary reinforcement. *J. Exp. Psychol.*, 24: 347.

MARTIN, A. 1945. A study of types of word-association in dementia praecox and manic-depressives. *J. Gen. Psychol.*, 33: 257.

MARTINO, G. 1939. The conditioned reflex of blinking. *J. Neurophysiol.*, 2: 173.

MASLOVA, N. P. 1958. Changes of EEG in neurotic patients (neurasthenia) awake, asleep and awakening. (Rus.) *Z. Vyss. Nerv. Dejat. Pavlova*, 8: 517.

MASSERMAN, J. H. 1939. An automatic apparatus for the central conditioning of small animals. *J. Comp. Psychol.*, 28: 201.

———. 1943. *Behavior and Neurosis.* Univ. Chicago Press.

———. 1951. La création des névroses expérimentales. *Psyche*, 6: 799.

MASSERMAN, J. H., *et al.* 1950. Effects of direct interrupted electroshock on experimental neuroses. *J. Nerv. Ment. Dis.*, 112: 384.

MASSERMAN, J. H., *et al.* 1944. Neurosis and alcohol: an experimental study. *Amer. J. Psychiat.*, 101: 389.

MASSERMAN, J. H., GROSS, Z., and PECHTEL, C. 1954. Abnormalities of behavior. *Ann. Rev. Psychol.*, 5: 263.

MASSERMAN, J. H., and PECHTEL, C. 1953. Conflict-engendered neurotic and psychotic behavior in monkeys. *J. Nerv. Ment. Dis.*, 118: 408.

———. 1956. How brain lesions affect normal and neurotic behavior: an experimental approach. *Amer. J. Psychiat.*, 112: 865.

———. 1956. Neurophysiologic and pharmacologic influences on experimental neuroses. *Ibid.*, 113: 510.

———. 1956. Normal and neurotic olfactory behavior in monkeys: a motion picture. *J. Nerv. Ment. Dis.*, 124: 518.

MASSERMAN, J. H., PECHTEL, C., and SCHREINER, L. 1953. The role of olfaction in normal and neurotic behavior in animals: preliminary report. *Psychosom. Med.*, 15: 396.

MASSERMAN, J. H., and SIEVER, P. W. 1944. Dominance, neurosis and aggression: an experimental study. *Psychosom. Med.*, 6: 7.

MASSERMAN, J. H., and YUM, K. S. 1946. An analysis of the influence of alcohol on experimental neuroses in cats. *Psychosom. Med.*, 8: 36.

MAYER-GROSS, W., SLATER, E., and ROTH, M. 1960. *Clinical Psychiatry.* Cassell.

MENZIES, R. 1937. Conditioned vasomotor responses in human subjects. *J. Psychol.*, 4: 75.

MERLIN, V. S. 1954. The characteristics of conditioned psychogalvanic reflexes in man. (Rus.) *Fiziol. Zh. SSSR*, 40: 155.

METZNER, C. A., and BAKER, L. E. 1939. The pupillary response conditioned to subliminal auditory stimuli: a control experiment. *Psychol. Bull.*, 36: 625.

MEYER, V., and GELDER, M. G. 1963. Behavior therapy and phobia disorders. *Brit. J. Psychiat.*, 109: 19.

MILEV, V. 1958. The clinical and experimental method in the study of hallucinations. (Rus.) *Z. Nevropat. Psikhiat. (Korsakoff)*, 58: 1465.

MILJUTIN, V. N. 1955. Disturbances in the dynamics of the cortical processes by hallucinations. (Rus.) *Z. Nevropat. Psikhiat. (Korsakoff)*, 55: 182.

MILLER, A. R. 1934. A failure to confirm Pavlov's hypothesis of external inhibition. *Amer. J. Physiol.*, 108: 605.

MILLER, J. 1939. The rate of conditioning of human subjects to single and multiple conditioned stimuli. *J. Gen. Psychol.*, 20: 399.

MILLER, S., and KONORSKI, J. 1928. Sur une forme particulière des réflexes conditionnels. *C.R. Soc. Biol.*, 99: 1155.

MINSKI, L. 1937. A note on some vasomotor disturbances in schizophrenia. *J. Ment. Sci.*, 83: 437.

MOELLER, C. G. 1950. Theoretical relationships among some measures of conditioning. *Proc. Nat. Acad. Sci.*, 36: 123.

———. 1954. The CS-US interval in GSR conditioning. *J. Exp. Psychol.*, 48: 162.

MONTGOMERY, K. C. 1951. An experimental investigation of reactive inhibition and conditioned inhibition. *J. Exp. Psychol.*, 41: 39.

MOORE, W. E. 1938. A conditioned reflex study of stuttering. *J. Speech Disorders*, 3: 163.

MORAVCSIK, E. E. 1911. Diagnostische Assoziations-untersuchungen. *Allg. Z. Psychiat.*, 68: 626.

MORISON, R. S., and DEMPSEY, E. W. 1942. A study of thalamocortical relations. *Amer. J. Physiol.*, 135: 281.

MORRELL, F., and JASPER, H. 1956. Electroencephalographic studies of the formation of temporary connections in the brain. *Electroencephalog. Clin. Neurophysiol.*, 8: 201.

MORRELL, F., NAQUET, R., and GASTAUT, H. 1957. Evolution of some electrical signs of conditioning. Part I. Normal cat and rabbit. *J. Neurophysiol.*, 20: 574.

MORRELL, F., ROBERTS, L., and JASPER, H. 1956. Effect of focal epileptogenic lesions and their ablation upon conditioned electrical responses of the brain in the monkey. *Electroencephalog. Clin. Neurophysiol.*, 8: 217.

MORRELL, F., and ROSS, M. 1953. Central inhibition in cortical conditioned reflexes, A.M.A. *Arch. Neurol. Psychiat.*, 70: 611.

MORUZZI, G., and MAGOUN, H. W. 1949. Brain stem reticular formation and activation of the EEG. *Electroencephalog. Clin. Neurophysiol.*, 1: 455.

MOTOKAWA, K. 1949. Electroencephalograms of man in the generalization of differentiation of conditioned reflexes. *Tohoku J. Exp. Med.*, 50: 225.

MOTOKAWA, K., and HUZIMORI, B. 1949. Electroencephalograms and conditioned reflexes. *Tohoku J. Exp. Med.*, 50: 215.

MOWRER, O. H. 1938. Preparatory set (expectancy)—a determinant in motivation and learning. *Psychol. Rev.*, 45: 62.

———. 1956. Two-factor learning theory reconsidered, with special reference to secondary reinforcement and the concept of habit. *Ibid.*, 63: 114.

———. 1960. *Learning Theory and Behavior.* Wiley.

MOWRER, O. H., and JONES, H. M. 1945. Habit strength as a function of the pattern of reinforcement. *J. Exp. Psychol.*, 35: 293.

MOWRER, O. H., and KEEHN, J. D. 1958. How are inter-trial "avoidance" responses reinforced? *Psychol. Rev.*, 65: 209.

MOWRER, O. H., and LAMOREAUX, R. R. 1946. Fear as an intervening variable in avoidance conditioning. *J. Comp. Psychol.*, 39: 29.

———. 1951. Conditioning and conditionality (discrimination). *Psychol. Rev.*, 58: 196.

MOYER, K. E. 1958. Effect of delay between training and extinction on the extinction of an avoidance response. *J. Comp. Physiol. Psychol.*, 51: 116.

MULLER-HEGEMANN, D. 1942. Assoziationsversuche mittels Silbenergänzung. *Nervenarzt*, 15: 389.

MULOTKOVA, I. A. 1957. Conditional reflexes to successive complex stimuli in oligophrenic patients. (Rus.) *Z. Vyss. Nerv. Dejat. Pavlova*, 7: 58.

MUNCIE, W. and GANTT, W. H. 1938. Effect on behavior of inhibition of different forms of excitation. *Amer. J. Physiol.*, 123: 152.

MUNN, N. L. 1939. The relative effectiveness of two conditioning procedures. *J. Gen. Psychol.*, 21: 119.

MURCHISON, C. 1934. *Handbook of General Experimental Psychology.* Clark Univ. Press.

MURPHY, G. 1921. A comparison of manic-depressive and dementia praecox cases by the free-association method. *Amer. J. Insan.*, 77: 545.

———. 1923. Types of word-association in dementia praecox, manic-depressives, and normal persons. *Amer. J. Psychiat.*, 2: 539.

MURPHY, J. V., and MILLER, R. E. 1957. Higher-order conditioning in the monkey. *J. Gen. Psychol.*, 56: 67.

MYERS, J. L. 1958. Secondary reinforcement: a review of recent experimentation. *Psychol. Bull.*, 55: 284.

NAGATY, M. O. 1951. The effect of reinforcement on closely following S-R conections. I. The effect of a backward conditioning procedure on the extinction of conditioned avoidance. *J. Exp. Psychol.*, 42: 239.

————. 1951. The effect of reinforcement on closely following S-R connections. II. Effect of Food reward immediately preceding performance of an instrumental conditioned response on extinction of that response. *Ibid.*, p. 333.

NATHAN, E. W. 1909. Uber die Assoziationen von Imbezillen und ihre diagnostische Verwertbarkeit. *Klin. Psych. Nerv. Krank.*, 4: 320.

NAUMENKO, A. I., and RAPPAPORT, A. I. 1940. Some characteristics of unconditioned and conditioned salivary activity of parotid and maxillary salivary glands. (Rus.) *Fiziol. Zh. SSSR*, 29: 501.

NOBLE, C. E. 1950. Conditioned generalization of the galvanic skin response to a subvocal stimulus. *J. Exp. Psychol.*, 40: 15.

NORRIS, EUGENIA B., and GRANT, D. A. 1948. Eyelid conditioning as effected by verbally induced inhibitory set and counter reinforcement. *Amer. J. Psychol.*, 61: 37.

NOTTERMAN, J. M. 1953. Experimental anxiety and a conditioned heart rate in human beings. *Trans. N.Y. Acad. Sci.*, 16: 24.

NYIRÖ, G. 1962. *Psychiatria*. Akademiai Kiado.

O'CONNOR, N., and RAWNSLEY, K. 1959. Two types of conditioning in psychotics and normals. *J. Abnorm. Soc. Psychol.*, 58: 157.

ODEGARD, O. 1930. The psychogalvanic reactivity in normals and in various psychopathic conditions. *Acta Psychiat. (Kbh.)*, 5: 55.

————. 1932. The psychogalvanic reactivity in affective disorders. *Brit. J. Med. Psychol.*, 12: 132.

OGIENKO, F. F. 1956. Vascular reactions in patients with various lesions of the central and peripheral nervous system. (Rus.) *Z. Vyss. Nerv. Dejat. Pavlova*, 6: 690.

OLDS, J. 1956. Runway and maze behavior controlled by basomedial forebrain stimulation in the rat. *J. Comp. Physiol. Psychol.*, 49: 507.

OLDS, J., KILLAM, K. F., and BACH-Y-RITA, P. 1956. Self-stimulation of the brain used as a screening method for tranquilizing drugs. *Science*, 124: 265.

OLDS, J., and MILNER, P. 1954. Positive reinforcement produced by electrical stimulation of septal area and other regions of rat brain. *J. Comp. Physiol. Psychol.*, 47: 419.

OLDS, J., and OLDS, M. E. 1958. Positive reinforcement produced by stimulating hypothalamus with iproniazid and other compounds. *Science*, 127: 1175.

OLDS, J., TRAVIS, R. P., and SCHWING, R. C. 1960. Topographic organization of hypothalamic self-stimulation functions. *J. Comp. Physiol. Psychol.*, 53: 23.

OSGOOD, C. E. 1953. Method and Theory in Experimental Psychology. Oxford Univ. Press.

OSWALD, I. 1962. Induction of illusory and hallucinatory voices with considerations of behavior therapy. *J. Ment. Sci.*, 108: 196.

OTIS, M. 1915. A study of association in defectives. *J. Educ. Psychol.*, 6: 271.

PAGE, H. A. 1955. The facilitation of experimental extinction by response prevention as a function of the acquisition of a new response. *J. Comp. Physiol. Psychol.*, 48: 14.

PAPEZ, J. W. 1958. Visceral brain, its component parts and their connections. *J. Nerv. Ment. Dis.*, 126: 40.

PARAMONOVA, N. P. 1957. Age peculiarities of interaction of the two signaling systems. (Rus.) *Z. Vyss. Nerv. Dejat. Pavlova*, 7: 651.

PAVLOV, B. V., and POVORINSKY, J. A. 1953. The interaction of the first and second signaling systems in the somnambulic phase of hypnosis. (Rus.) *Z. Vyss. Nerv. Dejat. Pavlova*, 3: 381.

PAVLOV, B. V., POVORINSKY, J. A., and BOBKOVA, V. V. 1955. The interaction of the first and second signaling systems in the somnambulic phase of hypnosis. (Rus.) *Z. Vyss. Nerv. Dejat. Pavlova*, 5: 11.

PAVLOV, I. P. 1902. *The Work of the Digestive Glands.* Translated by W. H. Thompson. Charles Griffin.

———. 1906. The scientific investigation of the psychical faculties or processes in the higher animals. *Lancet*, 2: 911.

———. 1927. *Conditioned Reflexes.* Translated by G. V. ANREP. Oxford Univ. Press.

———. 1928. *Conditioned Reflexes. An Investigation of the Physiological Activity of the Cerebral Cortex.* Translated and edited by G. V. ANREP. Oxford Univ. Press.

———. 1928. *Lectures on Conditioned Reflexes.* Translated by W. H. GANTT. International Publishers.

———. 1929. *Leçons sur le Travail des Hémisphères cérébraux.* Legrand.

———. 1932. *Les Reflexes Conditionnels.* Alcan.

———. 1932. Neuroses in man and animals. *J. Amer. Med. Assoc.*, 99: 1012.

———. 1932. The reply of a physiologist to a psychologist. *Psychol. Rev.*, 39: 91.

———. 1933. Esai d'une interpretation physiologique de l'hysterie. *Encéphale*, 28: 285.

———. 1934. An attempt at a physiological interpretation of obsessional neurosis and paranoia. *J. Ment. Sci.*, 80: 187.

———. 1941. *Conditioned Reflexes and Psychiatry.* Translated by W. H. GANTT. International Publishers.

———. 1941. *Lectures on Conditioned Reflexes.* Vol. II. *Conditioned Reflexes and Psychiatry.* Lawrance & Wishart.

————. 1953. *Samtliche Werke*. Akademie Verlag.

————. 1953. *Selected Papers*. (Hungarian.) Akademiai Kiado.

————. 1955. *Selected Works*. Translated by S. BELSKY; edited by J. GIBBONS. Foreign Language Publishing House.

————. 1956. *Mittwochkalloquien*. Akademie Verlag.

————. 1957. *Experimental Psychology and Other Essays*. Philosophical Library.

————. 1962. *Psychopathology and Psychiatry: Selected Works*. Translated by D. MYSHNE and S. BELSKY. Foreign Language Publishing House.

————. 1963. *Lectures on Conditioned Reflexes*. Translated by W. H. GANTT. Vol. I. International Publishers.

PAVLOVA, T. N. 1954. Changes in the higher nervous activity in operators of calculation machines during the working days. (Rus.) *Z. Vyss. Nerv. Dejat. Pavlova*, 4: 166.

PEIMER, I. A., UMAROV, M. B., and KHROMOV, N. A. 1954. Electrophysiological studies of psychasthenia and hysteria. (Rus.) *Z. Nevropat. Psikhiat. (Korsakoff)*, 54: 903.

PEN, R. M., and DZHAGAROV, M. A. 1936. The formation of conditional connections in hypnotic sleep. (Rus.) *Ark. Biol. Nauk*, 42: 77.

PENFIELD, W., and JASPER, H. 1954. *Epilepsy and the Functional Anatomy of the Human Brain*. Little, Brown.

PERELMAN, L. B. 1953. The methods of analyzing the functional conditions of the vaso-regulating mechanisms in hypertensive disease. (Rus.) *Z. Nevropat. Psikhiat. (Korsakoff)*, 53: 203.

PERKINS, C. C., JR. 1953. The relation between conditioned stimulus intensity and response strength. *J. Exp. Psychol.*, 46: 225.

PERMINOVA, I. D. 1953. The pseudohallucinatory syndrome of Kandinsky. (Rus.) *Z. Nevropat. Psikhiat. (Korsakoff)*, 53: 203.

PERVOV, L. G. 1956. Verbal method of determining the condition of higher nervous activity in man. (Rus.) *Z. Vyss. Nerv. Dejat. Pavlova*, 6: 329.

————. 1958. Complex studies of the higher nervous activity in hysteric patients. (Rus.) *Tr. Inst. Fiziol. Im. I.P. Pavlov*, 7: 225.

————. 1958. The higher nervous activity and the type of nervous system in hysteria studied with three experimental methods. *Ibid.*, p. 217.

————. 1958. Study of the higher nervous activity in patients suffering from hysteria. (Rus.) *Z. Vyss. Nerv. Dejat. Pavlova*, 8: 654.

PETERS, H. N., and MURPHREE, O. D. 1954. The conditional reflex in the chronic schizophrenic. *J. Clin. Psychol.*, 10: 126.

PETERSON, L. R. 1956. Variable delayed reinforcement. *J. Comp. Physiol. Psychol.*, 49: 232.

PFAFFMANN, C., and SCHLOSBERG, H. 1936. The conditioned knee jerk in psychotic and normal individuals. *J. Psychol.*, 1: 201.

PFEIFFER, C. C., and JENNEY, E. H. 1957. The inhibition of the conditional response and the counteraction of schizophrenia by muscarine stimulation of the brain. *Ann. N.Y. Acad. Sci.*, 66: 753.

PFEIFFER, C. C., RIOPELLE, A. J., SMITH, R. P., JENNEY, E. H., and WILLIAMS, H. L. 1957. Comparative study of the effect of meprobamate on the conditioned response, on strychnine and pentylenetetrazol thresholds, on the normal electroencephalogram and on polysynaptic reflexes. *Ann. N.Y. Acad. Sci.*, 67: 734.

PHILIP, B. R. 1947. Generalization and central tendency in the discrimination of a series of stimuli. *Can. J. Psychol.*, 1: 196.

PIAGET, JEAN. 1954. *Construction of Reality in the Child*. Basic Books.

PINTO, TERESA, and BROMILEY, R. B. 1950. A search for "spinal conditioning" and evidence that it can become a reflex. *J. Exp. Psychol.*, 40: 121.

PLATONOV, K. I. 1956. Psychotherapy of disturbed stereotypes of the higher nervous activity. (Rus.) *Z. Nevropat. Psikhiat. (Korsakoff)*, 56: 854.

———. 1959. *The Word as a Physiological and Therapeutic Factor*. Foreign Languages Publishing House.

PLESHKOVA, T. V. 1955. Conditional inhibition of the first and second signalling systems in hysteric neuroses. (Rus.) *Biull. éksp. Biol. Med.*, 39: 36.

———. 1957. Investigation of trace conditional inhibition in healthy persons and in patients suffering from neurasthenia. (Rus.) *Z. Vyss. Nerv. Dejat. Pavlova*, 7: 510.

PLOTICHER, A. I. 1955. Methodological variations in the study of conditional speech reactions of psychiatric patients. (Rus.) *Z. Vyss. Nerv. Dejat. Pavlova*, 5: 832.

POLTYREV, S. S. 1936. Die Rolle der Rinde und Subrindeknoten in der Bildung der bedingten Reflexe. *Z. Biol.*, 97: 180.

POLTYREV, S. S., and ZELIONY, G. P. 1930. Grosshirnrinde und Assoziationsfunction. *Z. Biol.*, 90: 157.

POPOV, C. 1956. Supramaximal inhibition studied by electroencephalographic methods on the rabbit. *Electroencephalog. Clin. Neurophysiol.*, 8: 728.

POPOV, E. A. 1955. The significance of the inhibitory phenomena in the clinic of psychiatric diseases. (Rus.) *Z. Vyss. Nerv. Dejat. Pavlova*, 5: 329.

———. 1957. The application of the Pavlovian theories in psychiatry. (Rus.) *Z. Nevropat. Psikhiat. (Korsakoff)*, 57: 673.

POPOV, N. A. 1923. Extinction of the investigatory reflex in the dog. (Rus.) *Fiziol. Zh. SSSR*, Vol. 3.

———. 1947. Etudes électroencéphalographiques du problème des réflexes conditionnés. *Année Psychol.*, 47: 97.

————. 1950. Etudes électroencéphalographiques du problème des réflexes conditionnés, III, IV. *J. Physiol.* (Paris), 42: 51.

POPPER, E. 1920. Uber schmerzgefühle bei Oligophrenen. *Neurol. Zbl.*, 39: 13.

PORTER, J. M., JR. 1938. Adaptation of the galvanic skin response. *J. Exp. Psychol.*, 23: 553.

————. 1938. Backward conditioning of the eyelid response. *Ibid.*, p. 403.

POSTMAN, L. 1947. The history and present status of the law of effect. *Psychol. Bull.*, 44: 489.

POVORINSKY, J. A., and TRAUGOTT, N. N. 1937. Some characteristics of the cortical dynamics in hypnotic sleep. (Rus.) *Ark. Biol. Nauk*, 44: 5.

PROKASY, W. F., JR. 1958. Extinction and spontaneous recovery of conditioned eyelid responses as a function of amount of acquisition and extinction training. *J. Exp. Psychol.*, 56: 319.

PROKASY, W. F., JR., GRANT, D. A., and MEYERS, N. A. 1958. Eyelid conditioning as a function of unconditioned stimulus intensity and intertrial interval. *J. Exp. Psychol.*, 55: 242.

PROKHOROVA, E. S. 1954. Some pathophysiological mechanisms of the hysteric paralysis. (Rus.) *Z. Vyss. Nerv. Dejat. Pavlova*, 4: 773.

PROKOFIEV, G., and ZELIONY, G. P. 1926. Des modes d'associations cérébrales chez l'homme et chez les animaux. *J. Psychol.* (Paris), 23: 1020.

PRONKO, N. H., and KELLOGG, W. N. 1942. The phenomenon of the muscle twitch in flexion conditioning. *J. Exp. Psychol.*, 31: 232.

PROSSER, C. L., and HUNTER, W. S. 1936. The extinction of startle responses and spinal reflexes in the white rat. *Amer. J. Physiol.*, 117: 609.

PROTOPOPOV, V. P. 1948. The somatic characteristics of manic-depressive psychoses. (Rus.) *Nevropat. i Psikhiat.*, 17: 57.

————. 1957. Problems of the manic-depressive psychosis. (Rus.) *Z. Nevropat. Psikhiat. (Korsakoff)*, 57: 1355.

RABIN, A. I., KING, G. F., and EHRMANN, J. C. 1955. Vocabulary performance of short-term and long-term schizophrenics. *J. Abnorm. Soc. Psychol.*, 50: 255.

RAJEVA, S. N. 1948. Studies of complex dynamic structures in patients with paranoid schizophrenia. (Rus.) *Tez. 18 Sov. Probl. Vyss. Nerv. Dejat. Ser. Patofiziol.*, 5: 157.

————. 1955. The influence of prolonged sleep on some disturbances of the cortical dynamics in hysteria. (Rus.) *Tr. Inst. Vyss. Nerv. Dejat. Ser. Patofiziol.*, 1: 230.

————. 1958. Characteristics of the interaction of the first and second signaling systems by the activation of pathodynamic structures in patients with paranoid schizophrenia. *Ibid.*, 5: 55.

RAYMOND, M. J. 1956. Case of fetishism treated by aversion therapy. *Brit. Med. J.*, 7: 854.

RAZRAN, G. H. S. 1930. Theory of conditioning and related phenomena. *Psychol. Rev.*, 37· 25.

————. 1933. Conditional responses in animals other than dogs. *Psychol. Bull.*, 30: 261.

————. 1933. Conditioned responses in children. *Arch. Psychol.*, 23: 148.

————. 1934. Conditional withdrawal response with shock as the conditioning stimulus in adult human subjects. *Psychol. Bull*, 31: 111.

————. 1938. Transposition of relational responses and generalization of conditioned responses. *Psychol. Rev.*, 45: 532.

————. 1939. Extinction, spontaneous recovery, and forgetting. *Amer. J. Psychol.*, 52: 100.

————. 1939. The law of effect or the law of qualitative conditioning. *Psychol. Rev.*, 46: 445.

————. 1939. A quantitative study of meaning by a conditioned salivary technique (semantic conditioning). *Science*, 90: 89.

————. 1939. Studies in configural conditioning. VI. Comparative extinction and forgetting of pattern and of single-stimulus conditioning. *J. Exp. Psychol.*, 24: 432.

————. 1949. Stimulus generalization of conditioned responses. *Psychol. Bull.*, 46: 337.

————. 1955. A direct laboratory comparison of Pavlovian conditioning and traditional associative learning. *J. Abnorm. Soc. Psychol.*, 51: 649.

————. 1955. A note on second-order-conditioning and secondary reinforcement. *Psychol. Rev.*, 62: 327.

————. 1955. Partial reinforcement of salivary CR's in adult human subjects: preliminary study. *Psychol. Rep.*, 1: 409.

————. 1955. Operant vs. classical conditioning. *Amer. J. Psychol.*, 68: 489.

————. 1956. Avoidant vs. unavoidant conditioning and partial reinforcement in Russian laboratories. *Amer. J. Psychol.*, 69: 127.

————. 1956. Backward conditioning. *Psychol. Bull.*, 53: 55.

————. 1956. Backward conditioning. *Ibid.*, p. 55.

————. 1956. Extinction re-examined and re-analyzed: a new theory. *Psychol. Rev.*, 63: 39.

————. 1957. The dominance-contiguity theory of the acquisition of classical conditioning. *Psychol. Bull.*, 54: 1.

REESE, W. G. 1953. Certain aspects of conditioning in the human. *Ann. N.Y. Acad. Sci.*, 56: 330.

REISER, L. A. 1955. Some peculiarities of the higher nervous activity in psychiatric patients studied by plethysmography. (Rus.) *Z. Vyss. Nerv. Dejat. Pavlova*, 5: 520.

REISS, B. F. 1946. Genetic changes in semantic conditioning. *J. Exp. Psychol.,* 36: 143.

REYNOLDS, B. 1945. The acquisition of a trace conditioned response as a function of the magnitude of the stimulus trace. *J. Exp. Psychol.,* 35: 15.

———. 1945. Extinction of trace conditioned responses as a function of the spacing of trials during the acquisition and extinction series. *Ibid.,* p. 81.

ROBINSON, J., and GANTT, W. H. 1947. The orienting reflex (questioning reaction): cardiac, respiratory, salivary and motor components. *Bull. Johns Hopkins Hosp.,* 80: 231.

ROESSLER, R. L., and BROGDEN, W. J. 1943. Conditioned differentiation of vasoconstriction to subvocal stimuli. *Amer. J. Psychol.,* 56: 78.

ROGER, A., SOKOLOV, E. N., and VORONINE, L. 1957. Le conditionnement moteur a l'état de vielle et pendant le sommeil. *Rev. Neurol.,* 96: 460.

ROHDE, M. 1911. Assoziationsvorgange bei Defektpsychosen. *Mschr. Psychiat. Neurol.,* 30: 272.

ROHRER, J. H. 1947. Experimental extinction as a function of the distribution of extinction trials and response strength. *J. Exp. Psychol.,* 37: 473.

ROKHLIN, L. 1958. *Soviet Medicine in the Fight against Mental Diseases.* Foreign Languages Publishing House.

RONCHEVSKY, S. P. 1928. Study on salivary secretory conditional reflexes of catatonics. (Rus.) *Nevropat i Psikhiat.,* 21: 340.

ROSANOFF, I. R., and ROSANOFF, A. J. 1913. A study of association in children. *Psychol. Rev.,* 20: 43.

ROSEN, V. H., and GANTT, W. H. 1943. Effect of metrazol convulsions on conditional reflexes in dogs. *Arch. Neurol. Psychiat.,* 50: 8.

ROSENBAUM, G. 1953. Stimulus generalization as a function of level of experimentally induced anxiety. *J. Exp. Psychol.,* 45: 35.

ROSS, L. E. 1959. The decremental effects of partial reinforcement during acquisition of the conditioned eyelid response. *J. Exp. Psychol.,* 57: 74.

ROTH, G. 1955. Die zerebralen Anfallsleiden im Elektroencephalogramm und im Jung'schen Assoziationstest. *Wien. Arch. Psychol. Psychiat. Neurol.,* 5: 206.

RUNQUIST, W. N., and ROSS, L. E. 1959. The relation between physiological measures of emotionality and performance in eyelid conditioning. *J. Exp. Psychol.,* 57: 329.

RUNQUIST, W. N., SPENCE, K. W., and STUBBS, D. W. 1958. Differential conditioning and intensity of the US. *J. Exp. Psychol.,* 55: 51.

RUSINOV, V. S. 1957. Electrophysiological investigations of the higher nervous activity. (Rus.) *Z. Vyss. Nerv. Dejat. Pavlova,* 7: 855.

RUSINOV, V. S., and RABINOVITCH, M. Y. 1958. Electroencephalographic researches in the laboratories and clinics of the Soviet Union. *Electroencephalog. Clin. Neurophysiol.*, Suppl., 8: 1.

RUTLEDGE, L. T., and DOTY, R. W. 1955. Differential action of chlorpromazine on conditional responses to peripheral versus direct cortical stimuli. *Fed. Proc.*, 14: 126.

SAIMOV, K. A. 1955. The interaction of the two signalling systems in phasic conditions. (Rus.) *Z. Nevropat. Psikhiat. (Korsakoff)*, 55: 176.

SAMOILOVA, Z. T. 1952. The influence of pharmacological and toxicological substances on conditional reflex activity. (Survey of studies of Soviet authors.) (Rus.) *Z. Vyss. Nerv. Dejat. Pavlova*, 2: 258.

SANDOMIRSKY, M. I. 1952. The clinical use of chronaximetry in psychiatric disorders. (Rus.) *Z. Nevropat. Psikhiat. (Korsakoff)*, 52: 24.

――――. 1955. Unconditional and conditional changes of the peripheral chronaxy in patients with infectious psychoses. *Ibid.*, 55: 759.

SAVCHUK, V. I. 1958. Unconditional vascular reflexes under various functional conditions of the cerebral cortex. (Rus.) *Z. Vyss. Nerv. Dejat. Pavlova*, 8: 804.

SCHAFER, R. 1945. Clinical evaluation of word association test. *Bull. Menninger Clin.*, 9: 84.

SCHEIBEL, M., *et al.* 1955. Convergence and interaction of afferent impulses on single units of reticular formation. *J. Neurophysiol.*, 18: 309.

SCHLOSBERG, H. 1928. A study of the conditioned patellar reflex. *J. Exp. Psychol.*, 11: 468.

――――. 1934. Conditioned responses in the white rat. *J. Genet. Psychol.*, 45: 303.

――――. 1936. Conditioned responses in the white rat. II. Conditioned responses based upon shock to the foreleg. *Ibid.*, 49: 107.

――――. 1937. The relationship between success and the laws of conditioning. *Psychol. Rev.*, 44: 379.

SEGAL, J. E. 1927. The elaboration of conditional reflexes and differentiation in oligophrenics. (Rus.) *Nevropat. i Psikhiat.*, 20: 535.

――――. 1953. The neurodynamics of vascular reactions in the hallucinatory-paranoid form of schizophrenia. (Rus.) *Z. Nevropat. Psikhiat. (Korsakoff)*, 53: 182.

――――. 1955. The neurodynamics of vascular reactions in the hallucinatory-paranoid form of schizophrenia. *Ibid.*, 55: 249.

SEIDEL, R. J. 1958. An investigation of the mediation process in preconditioning. *J. Exp. Psychol.*, 56: 220.

――――. 1959. A review of sensory preconditioning. *Psychol. Bull.*, 56: 58.

SEREDINA, M. I. 1953. Disturbances of the first and second signaling systems in chronic alcoholic hallucinosis. (Rus.) *Z. Vyss. Nerv. Dejat. Pavlova*, 3: 849.

———— 1953. Experimental and clinical studies of the interaction of the first and second signaling systems in delirium tremens. *Ibid.*, p. 99.

————. 1955. Disturbances of the first and second signaling systems in some forms of alcoholic hallucinations. (Rus.) *Tr. Inst. Vyss. Nerv. Dejat. Ser. Patofiziol.*, 1: 150.

————. 1955. Disturbances of the higher nervous activity in general paresis. *Ibid.*, p. 137.

————. 1955. Disturbances of the neurodynamics in anancastic neuroses. *Ibid.*, p. 67.

————. 1955. Experiences with pathogenetically based combined treatment of anancastic neuroses. *Ibid.*, p. 330.

————. 1955. The influence of caffein on the interaction of the first and second signaling systems in chronic alcoholic hallucinosis. *Ibid.*, p. 212.

————. 1958. Disturbances of the combined activity of the signaling systems in acute alcoholic hallucinosis. *Ibid.*, 5: 141.

————. 1958. Effect of sleep treatment on the combined activity of the first and second signaling systems in patients wih delirium tremens. *Ibid.*, p. 293.

SEREDINA, M. I., and POVORINSKY, J. A. 1955. The methods of studying motor conditional reflexes with verbal reinforcement. (Rus.) *Z. Nevropat. Psikhiat. (Korsakoff)*, 55: 871.

SERGEJEVA, K. A. 1953. Vascular conditional and unconditional reflexes in patients with obliterating endarteritis. (Rus.) *Z. Vyss. Nerv. Dejat. Pavlova*, 3: 865.

SERVIT, Z. 1955. Problems of the interaction of excitation and inhibition in the pathophysiology of epileptic seizures. (Rus.) *Z. Vyss. Nerv. Dejat. Pavlova*, 5: 474.

SETTLAGE, P. H., and HARLOW, H. F. 1936. Concerning the sensory pathway in the conditioned reflex. *J. Comp. Psychol.*, 22: 279.

SHAGASS, C., and JOHNSON, E. P. 1943. The course of acquisition of a conditioned response of the occipital alpha rhythm. *J. Exp. Psychol.*, 33: 201.

SHAKHNOVICH, A. R., and SHAKHNOVICH, V. R. 1954. The study of conditional pupillary reflexes in men without previous training. (Rus.) *Z. Nevropat. Psikhiat. (Korsakoff)*, 54: 313.

SHARGORODSKY, L. J. 1955. Some problems concerning the investigation methods and pathophysiology of unconditional vascular reflexes. (Rus.) *Z. Nevropat. Psikhiat. (Korsakoff)*, 55: 430.

SHARPLESS, S., and JASPER, H. 1956. Habituation of the arousal reaction. *Brain*, 79: 655.

SHATTOCK, F. M. 1950. The somatic manifestations of schizophrenia. *J. Ment. Sci.*, 96: 32.

SHEFFIELD, F. D. 1949. Hilgard's critique of Guthrie. *Psychol. Rev.*, 56: 284.

Sherrington, C. S. 1906. *The Integrative Action of the Nervous System.* Yale Univ. Press.

———. 1947. *The Integrative Action of the Nervous System.* Cambridge Univ. Press.

Shipley, W. C. 1933. An apparent transfer of conditioning. *J. Gen. Psychol.*, 8: 382.

———. 1935. Indirect conditioning. *Ibid.*, 12: 337.

Shumilina, A. I. 1956. Characteristics of the conditional reflex activity of dogs receiving aminazine. (Rus.) *Z. Nevropat. Psikhiat. (Korsakoff)*, 56: 116.

Shurrager, P. S., and Culler, E. 1938. Phenomena allied to conditioning in the spinal dog. *Amer. J. Physiol.*, 123: 186.

———. 1940. Conditioning in the spinal dog. *J. Exp. Psychol.*, 26: 133.

———. 1941. Conditioned extinction of a reflex in the spinal dog. *Ibid.*, 28: 287.

Shurrager, P. S., and Shurrager, H. C. 1941. Converting a spinal CR into a reflex. *J. Exp. Psychol.*, 29: 217.

———. 1950. Comment on "a search for spinal conditioning" and for evidence that it can become a reflex. *Ibid.*, 40: 135.

Shvedskaya, A. G. 1954. Characteristics of unconditional specific immunological reactions in schizophrenia. (Rus.) *Z. Nevropat. Psikhiat. (Korsakoff)*, 54: 741.

Sidman, M. 1953. Avoidance conditioning with brief shock and no exteroceptive warning signal. *Science*, 118: 157.

Silver, C. A., and Meyer, D. R. 1954. Temporal factors in sensory preconditioning. *J. Comp. Physiol. Psychol.*, 47: 57.

Sinkevich, Z. L. 1951. Disturbances in interaction of the first and second signaling systems in chronic alcoholism. (Rus.) *Z. Vyss. Nerv. Dejat. Pavlova*, 1: 608.

———. 1955. An attempt to investigate conditional inhibition in schizophrenics. (Rus.) *Tr. Inst. Vyss. Nerv. Dejat. Ser. Patofiziol.*, 1: 13.

Skinner, B. F. 1931. The concept of the reflex in the description of behavior. *J. Gen. Psychol.*, 5: 427.

———. 1932. On the rate of formation of a conditioned reflex. *Ibid.*, 7: 274.

———. 1933. The rate of establishment of a discrimination. *Ibid.*, 9: 302.

———. 1934. A discrimination without previous conditioning. *Proc. Nat. Acad. Sci.*, 20: 532.

———. 1934. The extinction of chained reflexes. *Ibid.*, p. 234.

———. 1935. A discrimination based upon a change in the properties of a stimulus. *J. Gen. Psychol.*, 12: 313.

———. 1935. Two types of conditioned reflex and a pseudo type. *Ibid.*, p. 66.

———. 1936. Conditioning and extinction and their relation to drive. *Ibid.*, 14: 296.

————. 1936. The effect on the amount of conditioning of an interval of time before reinforcement. *Ibid.*, p. 279.

————. 1936. A failure to obtain "disinhibition." *Ibid.*, p. 127.

————. 1936. The reinforcing effect of a differentiating stmulus. *Ibid.*, p. 263.

————. 1937. Two types of conditioned reflex: a reply to Konorski and Miller. *Ibid.*, 16: 272.

————. 1938. *The Behavior of Organisms: An Experimental Analysis.* Appleton-Century.

————. 1957. *Verbal Behavior.* Appleton-Century-Crofts.

SKINNER, B. F., SOLOMON, H. C., and LINDSLEY, O. R. 1954. A new method for the experimental analysis of the behavior of psychotic patients. *J. Nerv. Ment. Dis.*, 120: 403.

SLOAN, N., and JASPER, H. 1950. Identity of spreading depression and "suppression." *Electroencephalog. Clin. Neurophysiol.*, 2: 59.

SMETANNIKOV, P. G. 1957. On the influence of caffein on the higher nervous activity of patients with syndromes of amentia after infections and intoxications. (Rus.) *Z. Nevropat. Psikhiat.*, *(Korsakoff)*, Suppl., 57: 59.

SMIRNOV, D. A. 1953. The word experiment in medical practice. (Rus.) *Z. Vyss. Nerv. Dejat., Pavlova*, 3: 408.

SMITH, K. Conditioning as an artifact. *Psychol. Rev.*, 61: 217.

SMITH, S., and GUTHRIE, E. R. 1921. *General Psychology in Terms of Behavior.* Appleton-Century-Crofts.

SOKOLOV, E. N., and PARAMONOVA, N. P. 1956. On the role of orientative reflexes in establishing motor conditional reactions in man. (Rus.) *Z. Vyss. Nerv. Dejat. Pavlova*, 6: 702.

SOKOLOVA, G. S. 1958. Conditional traced eyelid reflexes in neurotics with depressive syndromes. (Rus.) *Tez. 18 Sov. Probl. Vyss. Nerv. Dejat.*, 3: 136.

————. 1958. Traced conditional eyelid reflexes in healthy persons and neurotic patients. (Rus.) *Tr. Inst. Fiziol. Im. I.P. Pavlov*, 7: 239.

SOLOMON, R. L. 1948. Effort and extinction rate: a confirmation. *J. Comp. Physiol. Psychol.*, 41: 93.

SPELT, D. K. 1938. Conditioned responses in the human fetus in utero. *Psychol. Bull.*, 35: 712.

————. 1948. The conditioning of the human fetus in utero. *J. Exp. Psychol.*, 38: 338.

SPENCE, K. W. 1944. The nature of theory construction in contemporary psychology. *Psychol. Rev.*, 51: 47.

————. 1947. The role of secondary reinforcement in delayed-reward learning. *Ibid.*, 54: 1.

————. 1948. The postulates and methods of behaviorism. *Ibid.*, 55: 67.

————. 1952. The nature of the response in discrimination learning. *Ibid.*, 59: 89.

————. 1953. Learning and performance in eyelid conditioning as a function of the intensity of the UCS. *J. Exp. Psychol.*, 45: 57.

————. 1956. *Behavior Theory and Conditioning.* Yale Univ. Press.

SPENCE, K. W., and BEECROFT, R. S. 1954. Differential conditioning and level of anxiety. *J. Exp. Psychol.*, 48: 399.

SPENCE, K. W., BERGMAN, G., and LIPPITT, R. A. 1950. A study of simple learning under irrelevant motivational-reward conditions. *J. Exp. Psychol.*, 40: 539.

SPENCE, K. W., and FARBER, I. E. 1953. Conditioning and extinction as a function of anxiety. *J. Exp. Psychol.*, 45: 116.

————. 1954. The relation of anxiety to differential eyelid conditioning. *Ibid.*, 47: 127.

SPENCE, K. W., FARBER, I. E., and TAYLOR, ELAINE. 1954. The relation of electric shock and anxiety to level of performance in eyelid conditioning. *J. Exp. Psychol.*, 48: 404.

SPENCE, K. W., GOODRICH, K. P., and Ross, L. E. 1959. Performance in differential conditioning and discrimination learning as a function of hunger and relative response frequency. *J. Exp. Psychol.*, 58: 8.

SPENCE, K. W., HAGGARD, D. F., and Ross, L. E. 1958. Intrasubject conditioning as a function of the intensity of the unconditioned stimulus. *Science*, 128: 774.

————. 1958. US intensity and the associative (habit) strength of the eyelid CR. *J. Exp. Psychol.*, 55: 404.

SPENCE, K. W., and NORRIS, E. B. 1950. Eyelid conditioning as a function of the inter-trial interval. *J. Exp. Psychol.*, 40: 716.

SPENCE, K. W., and Ross, L. E. 1959. A methodological study of the form and latency of eyelid responses in conditioning. *J. Exp. Psychol.*, 58: 376.

SPENCE, K. W., and TAYLOR, JANET A. 1951. Anxiety and strength of U.S. as determiners of the amount of eyelid conditioning. *J. Exp. Psychol.*, 42: 183.

————. 1953. The relation of conditional response strength to anxiety in normal, neurotic, and psychotic subjects. *Ibid.*, 45: 265.

SPIVAK, L. I. 1953. Patellar reflex changes in depressive and hypomanic states. (Rus.) *Z. Nevropat. Psikhiat. (Korsakoff)*, 53: 422.

SPOONER, A., and KELLOGG, W. N. 1947. The backward-conditioning curve. *Amer. J. Psychol.*, 60: 321.

STANISHEVSKAYA, N. N. 1954. Clinical and pathophysiological studies of schizophrenics treated with tissue, sleep and insulin. (Rus.) *Z. Vyss. Nerv. Dejat. Pavlova*, 4: 184.

————. 1957. Some peculiarities of the vascular, motor and respiratory components of reflex activity in patients suffering from schizophrenia. *Ibid.*, 7: 683.

STANLEY, W. C. 1952. Extinction as a function of the spacing of extinction trials. *J. Exp. Psychol.*, 43: 249.

STARZL, T. E., TAYLOR, C. W., and MAGOUN, H. W. 1951. Collateral afferent excitation of reticular formation of brain stem. *J. Neurophysiol.*, 14: 479.

STECKLE, L. C. 1936. Two additional attempts to condition the pupillary reflex. *J. Gen. Psychol.*, 15: 369.

STECKLE, L. C., and RENSHAW, S. 1934. An investigation of the conditioned iridic reflex. *J. Gen. Psychol.*, 11: 3.

STENGEL, E., OLDHAM, A. J., and EHRENBERG, A. S. C. 1955. Reactions to pain in various abnormal mental states. *J. Ment. Sci.*, 101: 52.

STOCKER, A. 1953. La névrose considéré comme un réflexe conditionnel "sui generis." *Encéphale*, 42: 455.

STORM VAN LEEUWEN, W., BEKKERING, D. H., and KAMP, A. 1958. Some results obtained with the EEG Spectrograph. *Electroencephalog. Clin. Neurophysiol.*, 10: 563.

STRONG, E. K. 1913. A comparison between experimental data and clinical results in manic-depressive insanity. *Amer. J. Psychol.*, 24: 66.

SWITZER, S. A. 1930. Backward conditioning of the lid reflex. *J. Exp. Psychol.*, 13: 76.

————. 1933. Disinhibition of the conditioned galvanic skin response. *J. Gen. Psychol.*, 9: 77.

————. 1935. The effect of caffeine on experimental extinction of conditioned reactions. *Ibid.*, 12: 78.

TAFFEL, C. 1955. Anxiety and the conditioning of verbal behavior. *J. Abnorm. Soc. Psychol.*, 51: 496.

TARANSKAYA, A. D. 1956. Effect of atropine and pilocarpine on the conditional reflexes in mentally deranged patients. (Rus.) *Z. Vyss. Nerv. Dejat. Pavlova*, 6: 100.

TATARENKO, N. P. 1928. Reflex mechanisms in schizophrenics. (Rus.) *Vracheb. Delo.*, 3: 217.

————. 1954. The pathophysiology of schizophrenia. (Rus.) *Z. Nevropat. Psikhiat. (Korsakoff)*, 54: 710.

————. 1954. The pupillary components of the orienting reaction and the aspects of its clinical use. *Ibid.*, p. 153.

————. 1955. Some controversial problems in the theories of schizophrenia. *Ibid.*, 55: 837.

————. 1956. The significance of studying the orienting reflex in the psychiatric clinic. (Rus.) *Z. Vyss. Nerv. Dejat. Pavlova*, 6: 360.

————. 1958. Principles and methods of evaluating the effects of treatment in schizophrenia. (Rus.) *Z. Nevropat. Psikhiat. (Korsakoff)*, 58: 722.

TAYLOR, JANET A. 1951. The relationship of anxiety to the conditioned eyelid response. *J. Exp. Psychol.*, 41: 81.

————. 1956. Level of conditioning and intensity of the adapting stimulus. *Ibid.*, 51: 127.

TEICHNER, W. H. 1952. Experimental extinction as a function of the intertrial intervals during conditioning and extinction. *J. Exp. Psychol.*, 44: 170.

TEN CATE, J. 1934. Können die bedingten Reactionen sich auch ausserhalb der Grosshirnrinde bilden? *Arch Néerl. Physiol.*, 19: 469.

———. 1934. Die Pupillenverengerung, als bedingter Reflex auf akustische Reize und ihre Beziehung zu der Grosshirnrinde. *Ibid.*, p. 417.

TENDLER, A. D. 1933. Associative tendencies in psychoneurotics. *Psychol. Clin.*, 22: 108.

———. 1945. Significant features of disturbance in free association. *J. Psychol.*, 20: 65.

THORNDIKE, E. L. 1898. Animal intelligence: an experimental study of the associative processes in animals. *Psychol. Monogr.*, 2: 8.

———. 1909. Darwin's contribution to psychology. *Univ. Calif. Chron.*, 12: 65.

———. 1911. *Animal Intelligence*. Macmillan.

TOLMAN, E. C. 1922. A new formula for behaviorism. *Psychol. Rev.*, 29: 44.

———. 1926. A behavioristic theory of ideas. *Ibid.*, 33: 352.

———. 1927. A behaviorist's definition of consciousness. *Ibid.*, 34: 433.

———. 1932. *Purposive Behavior in Animals and Men*. Appleton-Century.

———. 1936. Sign-gestalt or conditioned reflex? *Psychol. Rev.*, 43: 258.

TORCHINSKAYA, V. A. 1954. Problems of the pathophysiology of manic-depressive psychosis. (Rus.) *Z. Nevropat. Psikhiat. (Korsakoff)*, 54: 934.

TRAUGOTT, N. N. 1952. The investigative methods of the interaction of the signaling systems in the psychiatric clinic. (Rus.) *Z. Nevropat. Psikhiat. (Korsakoff)*, 52: 3.

TRAUGOTT, N. N., and CHISTOVICH, A. S. 1952. Problems concerning the higher nervous activity in chronic delusional states (paraphrenia). (Rus.) *Tr. Inst. Fiziol. Im. I.P. Pavlov.*, 1: 413.

TROFIMOV, N. M. 1955. Characteristics of the conditional reflex activity in different stages of mental deficiency. (Rus.) *Z. Vyss. Nerv. Dejat. Pavlova*, 5: 358.

TRUNOVA, M. M. 1958. Disturbances of the combined activity of the signaling systems in anancastic neuroses and psychasthenia. (Rus.) *Tr. Inst. Vyss. Nerv. Dejat. Ser. Patofiziol.*, 5: 177.

TUSHINSKAYA, M. M. 1956. Study of higher nervous activity in patients affected with neuroses of the neurasthenia type. (Rus.) *Z. Vyss. Nerv. Dejat. Pavlova*, 6: 108.

ULETT, G. 1955. Discussion of Morrell, F., and Jasper, H. Conditioning of cortical electrical activity in the monkey. *Electroencephalog. Clin. Neurophysiol.*, 7: 461.

USOV, A. G. 1955. A complex method for the study of the higher nervous activity in the normal and the mentally sick. (Rus.) *Z. Vyss. Nerv. Dejat. Pavlova.*, 5: 825.

————. 1955. Experimental data on problems of the oxygen effect on the higher nervous activity of old persons. *Ibid.*, p. 351.

————. 1955. Studies of the induced interrelations of the signaling systems in healthy old persons and in patients with senile psychoses. *Ibid.*, p. 807.

VALENTINE, MAX. 1962. *An Introduction to Psychiatry*. E. & S. Livingstone.

VERPLANCK, W. S. 1956. The operant conditioning of human operant behavior. *Psychol. Bull.*, 53: 70.

VIGOUROUX, R., GASTAUT, H., and BADIER, M. 1951. Les formes expérimentales de l'épilepsie: provocation des principales manifestations cliniques de l'épilepsie dite temporal, par stimulation des structures rhinencéphaliques chez le chat anesthésié. *Rev. Neurol.*, 85: 505.

VINAR, O. 1958. Analogien zwischen schizophrenen Erkrankungen und der LSD-Psychose. *Psychol. Neurol. Med. Psychol.*, 10: 162.

VOEKS, VIRGINIA W. 1954. Acquisition of S-R connections: a test of Hull's and Guthrie's theories. *J. Exp. Psychol.*, 47: 137.

————. 1955. Gradual strengthening of S-R connections or increasing number of S-R connections. *J. Psychol.*, 39: 289.

VOTAVA, ZDENEK (ed.). 1963. *Psychopharmacological Methods*. Pergamon.

VALTER, W. G. 1950. The functions of the electrical rhythms in the brain. *J. Ment. Sci.*, 96: 1.

————. 1953. *The Living Brain*. Duckworth.

————. 1957. Conditionnement et réactivité. *Electroencephalog. Clin. Neurophysiol.*, Suppl. 6.

WALTER, W. G., and SHIPTON, H. W. 1951. A new toposcopic display system. *Electroencephalog. Clin. Neurophysiol.*, 3: 281.

WATSON, J. B. 1913. Psychology as the behaviorist views it. *Psychol. Rev.*, 20: 158.

————. 1916. Behavior and the concept of mental disease. *J. Philos. Psychol. Sci. Method.*, 13: 589.

————. 1916. The place of the conditioned reflex in psychology. *Psychol. Rev.*, 23: 89.

————. 1919. *Psychology from the Standpoint of a Behaviorist*. Lippincott.

————. 1925. *Behaviorism*. Norton.

WATSON, J. B., and RAYNER, R. 1920. Conditioned emotional reactions. *J. Exp. Psychol.*, 3: 1.

WEBER, H., and WENDT, G. R. 1942. Conditioning of eyelid closures with various conditions of reinforcement. *J. Exp. Psychol.*, 30: 114.

WEDELL, C. H., TAYLOR, F. V., and SKOLNICK, A. 1940. An attempt to condition the pupillary response. *J. Exp. Psychol.*, 27: 517.

WEINSTOCK, S. 1954. Resistance to extinction of a running response following partial reinforcement under widely spaced trials. *J. Comp. Physiol. Psychol.*, 47: 318.

————. 1958. Acquisition and extinction of a partially reinforced running response at a 24-hour intertrial interval. *J. Exp. Psychol.*, 56: 151.

WELCH, L. 1955. The relationship between conditioning and higher learning. *J. Gen. Psychol.*, 53: 221.

WELCH, L., and KUBIS, J. 1947. The effect of anxiety and the conditioning rate, and stability of the P.G.R. *J. Psychol.*, 23: 83.

WELLS, F. L. 1919. Autistic mechanisms in association reaction. *Psychol. Rev.*, 26: 376.

WELLS, HARRY K. 1963. *Ivan P. Pavlov: Toward a Scientific Psychology and Psychiatry.* International Publishers.

WENDT, G. R. 1930. An analytical study of the conditioned kneejerk. *Arch. Psychol.*, 19: 123.

WENDT, H. 1956. Schlaftherapie und zweites Signalsystem. *Z. Psychosom. Med.*, 2: 215.

WENGER, M. A. 1936. An investigation of conditioned responses in human infants. *Univ. Iowa Stud. Child Welfare*, 12: 7.

WENGER, M. A., JONES, F. N., and JONES, H. J. 1956. *Physiological Psychology.* Holt.

WHATMORE, G. B., and KLEITMAN, N. 1946. The role of sensory and motor cortical projections in the escape and avoidance conditioning in dogs. *Amer. J. Physiol.*, 146: 282.

WHATMORE, G. B., MORGAN, E. A., and KLEITMAN, N. 1946. The influence of avoidance conditioning on the course of non-avoidance conditioning in dogs. *Amer. J. Physiol.*, 145: 432.

WHITE, C. T., and SCHLOSBERG, H. 1952. Degree of conditioning of the G.S.R. as a function of the period of delay. *J. Exp. Psychol.*, 43: 357.

WHITE, R. P., and WESTERTEHE, E. J. 1961. Differences in central anticholinergic actions of phenothiazine derivatives. *Exp. Neurology*, 4: 317.

WHITE, S. H. 1958. Generalization of an instrumental response with variation in two attributes of the CS. *J. Exp. Psychol.*, 56: 339.

WICKENS, D. D. 1938. The transference of conditioned excitation and conditioned inhibition from one muscle group to the antagonistic muscle group. *J. Exp. Psychol.*, 22: 101.

————. 1939. The simultaneous transfer of conditioned excitation and conditioned inhibition. *Ibid.*, 24: 332.

————. 1939. A study of voluntary and involuntary finger-conditioning. *Ibid.*, 25: 127.

————. 1943. Studies of response generalization in conditioning. I. Stimulus generalization during response generalization. *Ibid.*, 33: 221.

————. 1948. Stimulus identity as related to response specificity and response generalization. *Ibid.*, 38: 389.

WICKENS, D. D., and BRIGGS, G. E. 1951. Mediated stimulus generalization as a factor in sensory preconditioning. *J. Exp. Psychol.*, 42: 197.

WICKENS, D. D., and WICKENS, CAROL D. 1940. A study of conditioning in the neonate. *J. Exp. Psychol.*, 26: 94.

————. 1942. Some factors related to pseudo-conditioning. *Ibid.*, 31: 518.

WILLIAMS, K. A. 1929. The reward value of a conditioned stimulus. *Univ. Calif. Publ. Psychol.*, 4: 31.

WILLIAMS, S. B. 1938. Resistance to extinction as a function of the number of reinforcements. *J. Exp. Psychol.*, 23: 506.

WINNICK, WILMA A., and HUNT, J. McV. 1951. The effect of an extra stimulus upon strength of response during acquisition and extinction. *J. Exp. Psychol.*, 41: 205.

WOLFE, J. B. 1934. The effect of delayed reward upon learning in the white rat. *J. Comp. Psychol.*, 17: 1.

WOLFLE, HELEN M. 1930. Time factors in conditioning finger-withdrawal. *J. Gen. Psychol.*, 4: 372.

————. 1932. Conditioning as a function of the interval between the conditioned and the original stimulus. *Ibid.*, 7: 80.

WOLPE, J. 1958. *Psychotherapy by Reciprocal Inhibition.* Stanford Univ. Press.

WOODWORTH, ROBERT S., and SCHLOSBERG, H. 1938, 1956. *Experimental Psychology.* Holt.

YACORZYNSKI, G. K., and GUTHRIE, E. R. 1937. A comparative study of involuntary and voluntary conditioned responses. *J. Gen. Psychol.*, 16: 235.

YAKOVLEVA, E. K. 1952. Characteristics of the electrical activity of the cerebral cortex in anancastic neuroses. (Rus.) *Z. Nevropat. Psikhiat. (Korsakoff)*, 52: 20.

————. 1957. The problem of experimental neuroses. (Rus.) *Z. Vyss. Nerv. Dejat. Pavlova*, 7: 841.

YERKES, R. M., and MORGULIS, S. 1909. The method of Pavlov in animal psychology. *Psychol. Bull.*, 6: 257.

YOSHII, N. 1957. Principes methadologiques de l'investigation électroencéphalographique du comportement conditionné. *Electroencephalog. Clin. Neurophysiol.*, Suppl. 6, p. 75.

YOSHII, N., and HOCKADAY, W. J. 1958. Conditioning of frequency characteristic repetitive EEG response with intermittent photic stimulation. *Electroencephalog. Clin. Neurophysiol.*, 10: 487.

YOSHII, N., PRUVOT, P., and GASTAUT, H. 1957. Electroencephalographic activity of the mesencephalic reticular formation during conditioning in the cat. *Electroencephalog. Clin. Neurophysiol.*, 9: 595.

YOUNG, F. A. 1954. An attempt to obtain pupillary conditioning with infrared photography. *J. Exp. Psychol.*, 48: 62.

————. 1958. Studies of pupillary conditioning. *Ibid.*, 55: 97.

YOUNG, P. T. 1936. *Motivation of Behavior.* Wiley.

YOUTZ, R. E. P. 1938. The change in time of a Thorndikean response in the rat. *J. Exp. Psychol.*, 23: 128.

————. 1938. Reinforcement, extinction, and spontaneous recovery in a non-Pavlovian reaction. *Ibid.*, 22: 305.

————. 1939. The weakening of one Thorndikean response following the extinction of another. *Ibid.*, 24: 294.

ZEAMAN, D. 1949. Response latency as a function of the amount of reinforcement. *J. Exp. Psychol.*, 39: 466.

ZEAMAN, D., and HOUSE, BETTY J. 1951. The growth and decay of reactive inhibition as measured by alternation behavior. *J. Exp. Psychol.*, 41: 177.

ZELIONY, G. P. 1929. Effets de l'ablation des hémisphères cérébraux. *Rev. Med.*, 46: 191.

ZENER, K. 1937. The significance of behavior accompanying conditioned salivary secretion for theories of the conditioned response. *Amer. J. Psychol.*, 50: 384.

ZIMMERMAN, D. W. 1957. Durable secondary reinforcement: method and theory. *Psychol. Rev.*, 64: 373.

ZNAMENSKY, V. V. 1953. The problems of the strength of reactivity in schizophrenia. (Rus.) *Z. Nevropat. Psikhiat. (Korsakoff)*, 53: 753.

ZURABASHVILI, A. D. 1952. The neurodynamic analysis of psychopathological phenomena. (Rus.) *Z. Vyss. Nerv. Dejat. Pavlova*, 2: 393.

————. 1955. Some data about the work signalization. (Rus.) *Z. Nevropat. Psikhiat. (Korsakoff)*, 55: 805.

LIST OF JOURNALS

Acta Neurol. Latinoamer.	Acta Neurologica Latinoamerica
Acta Pharmacol. Toxicol.	Acta pharmacologica et toxicologica
Acta Physiol. Hung.	Acta Physiologica Academeae Scientarium Hungaricae
Acta Physiol. Pharmacol. Néerl.	Acta physiologica et pharmacologica Néerlandica
Acta Psychiat.	Acta Psychiatrica et neurologica
Acta Psychiat. Scand.	Acta Psychiatrica Scandinavica
Acta Psychol.	Acta Psychologica
Allg. Z. Psychiat.	Allgemeine Zeitschrift für Psychiatrie
Amer. J. Dis. Child.	American Journal of Diseases of Children
Amer. J. Insan.	American Journal of Insanity
Amer. J. Ment. Defic.	American Journal of Mental Deficiency
Amer. J. Orthopsychiat.	American Journal of Orthopsychiatry
Amer. J. Physiol.	American Journal of Physiology
Amer. J. Psychiat.	American Journal of Psychiatry
Amer. J. Psychol.	American Journal of Psychology
Amer. Rev. Physiol.	American Review of Physiology
Angiology	Angiology
Ann. N.Y. Acad. Sci.	Annals of the New York Academy of Science
Année Psychol.	Année psychologique (Paris)
Ann. Méd. Psychol.	Annales médico-psychologiques
Ann. Rev. Physiol.	Annual Review of Physiology
Ann. Rev. Psychol.	Annual Review of Psychology
Arch. Int. Pharmacodyn.	Archives internationales de pharmacodynamie (et de therapie)
Arch. Néerl. Physiol.	Archives néerlandaises de physiologie de l'homme et des animaux
Arch. Neurol. Psychiat.	Archives of Neurology and Psychiatry
Arch. Psychiat. Nervenkr.	Archiv für Psychiatrie und Nervenkrankheiten
Arch. Psychol.	Archives of Psychology
Ark. Biol. Nauk	Arkhiv Biologicii Nauk
Assoc. Res. Nerv. Ment. Dis. Proc.	Association for Research in Nervous and Mental Disease, Proceedings

Biochem. Pharm.	*Biochemical Pharmacology*
Bjul. éksp. Biol. Med.	*Bjulleten éksperimental noi biologii i meditsiny*
Brain	*Brain: A Journal of Neurology*
Brit. J. Med. Psychol.	*British Journal of Medical Psychology*
Brit. J. Psychiat.	*British Journal of Psychiatry*
Brit. J. Psychol.	*British Journal of Psychology*
Brit. Med. J.	*British Medical Journal*
Bruxelles Psychol. Franç.	*Bruxelles Psychologie Française*
Bull. Exp. Biol. Med.	*Bulletin of Experimental Biology and Medicine*
Bull. Johns Hopkins Hosp.	*Bulletin of the Johns Hopkins Hospital*
Bull. Menninger Clin.	*Bulletin of the Menninger Clinic*
Bull. World Health Organ.	*Bulletin of the World Health Organization*
Can. J. Psychol.	*Canadian Journal of Psychology*
Can. Med. Assoc. J.	*Canadian Medical Association Journal*
Child Developm.	*Child Development*
Comp. Psychol. Monogr.	*Comparative Psychology Monographs*
C.R. Soc. Biol.	*Comptes rendus des séances de la Societé de biologie*
Dis. Nerv. Syst.	*Diseases of the Nervous System*
Dokl. Akad. Nauk SSSR	*Doklady Akademii Nauk SSSR*
Electroencephalog. Clin. Neurophysiol.	*Electroencephalography and Clinical Neurophysiology*
Encéphale	*Encéphale (et hygiène mentale)*
Exp. Neurology	*Experimental Neurology*
Fed. Proc.	*Federation Proceedings*
Fiziol. Zh. SSSR	*Fiziologicheskii Zhurnal SSSR Imeni I.M. Sechenova*
Iowa Acad. Sci.	*Iowa Academy of Science*
Jb. Kinderheilk.	*Jahrbuch für Kinderheilkunde und physische Erziehung*
J. Abnorm. Soc. Psychol.	*Journal of Abnormal and Social Psychology*
J. Amer. Med. Assoc.	*Journal of the American Medical Association*
J. Clin. Exp. Psychopathol.	*Journal of Clinical and Experimental Psychopathology and Quarterly Review of Psychiatry*
J. Clin. Psychol.	*Journal of Clinical Psychology*
J. Comp. Physiol. Psychol.	*Journal of Comparative and Physiological Psychology*
J. Comp. Psychol.	*Journal of Comparative Psychology*
J. Educ. Psychol.	*Journal of Educational Psychology*
J. Exp. Psychol.	*Journal of Experimental Psychology*

J. Gen. Psychol.	*Journal of General Psychology*
J. Genet. Psychol.	*Journal of Genetic Psychology*
J. Ment. Sci.	*Journal of Mental Science*
J. Mt. Sinai Hosp.	*Journal of the Mount Sinai Hospital*
J. Nerv. Ment. Dis.	*Journal of Nervous and Mental Disease*
J. Neurophysiol.	*Journal of Neurophysiology*
J. Neurosurg.	*Journal of Neurosurgery*
J. Personality	*Journal of Personality*
J. Pharmacol.	*Journal of Pharmacology*
J. Phil. Psychol. Sci. Methods	*Journal of Philosophy, Psychology and Scientific Methods*
J. Physiol.	*Journal of Physiology*
J. Physiol. (Paris)	*Journal de physiologie* (Paris)
J. Psychol.	*Journal of Psychology*
J. Psychol. (Paris)	*Journal de psychologie* (Paris)
J. Psychosom. Res.	*Journal of Psychosomatic Research*
J. Speech Disord.	*Journal of Speech Disorders*
Klin. Med.	*Klinicheskaia Meditsina*
Klin Psych. Nerv. Krank.	*Klinik für psychische und nervöse Krankheiten*
Klin. Wschr.	*Klinische Wochenschrift*
Lancet	*Lancet*
Med. J. Osaka Univ.	*Medical Journal of Osaka University*
Mschr. Psychiat. Neurol.	*Monatschrift für Psychiatrie und Neurologie*
Nervenarzt	*Nervenarzt*
Neurol. Neurochir. Psychiat. Polska	*Neurologia, Neurochirugia i Psychiatrie Polska*
Neurol. Zb.	*Neurologisches Zentralblatt*
Nevropat. i Psikhiat.	*Nevropatologii i Psikhiatrii*
Nord. Psykiat. Medlemsbl.	*Nordisk psykiatrisk Medlemsblad*
Phil. Rev.	*Philosophical Review*
Physiol. Bohemosl.	*Physiologia Bohemoslovenica*
Proc. Nat. Acad. Sci.	*Proceedings of the National Academy of Sciences*
Proc. Roy. Soc.	*Proceedings of the Royal Society of Medicine*
Prog. Psychother.	*Progress in Psychotherapy*
Psikhiat. Klin. Probl. Patol. Vyss. Nerv. Dejat.	*Psikhiatrii Klinicheskai Problemy Patologii Vysshei Nervnoi Dejatel*
Psikhiat. Nevropatol. éksp. Psikol.	*Psikhiatrii Nevropatologii éksperimental Psikologii*
Psyche	*Psyche: revue internationale de psychoanalyse*

Psychiat. Neurol. Med. Psychol.	*Psychiatrie, Neurologie und medizinische Psychologie*
Psychiat. Res. Rep.	*Psychiatric Research Reports*
Psychol. Arb.	*Psychologische Arbeiten*
Psychol. Bull.	*Psychological Bulletin*
Psychol. Clin.	*Psychological Clinic*
Psychol. Monogr.	*Psychological Monographs*
Psychol. Rep.	*Psychological Reports*
Psychol. Rev.	*Psychological Review*
Psychosom. Med.	*Psychosomatic Medicine*
Publ. Beritashvili Inst. Fiziol.	*Publikatsii Beritashvili Instituta Fiziologicheskii*
Publ. Pavlov Fiziol. Inst.	*Publikatsii Pavlov Fiziologicheskii Instituta*
Rev. Méd.	*Revue de Médicine*
Rev. Neurol.	*Revue neurologique*
Schweiz. Arch. Neurol. Psychiat.	*Schweizer Archiv für Neurologie und Psychiatrie*
Science	*Science*
South. Med. J.	*Southern Medical Journal*
Studi si Cercet. Neurol.	*Studii si cercetari de neurologie*
Tez. 18 Sov. Probl. Vyss. Nerv. Dejat.	*Tezisy 18 Sovetsky Problemy Vysshei Nervnoi Dejatel'nosti*
Tohoku J. Exp. Med.	*Tohoku Journal of Experimental Medicine*
Trans. Amer. Neurol. Assoc.	*Transactions of the American Neurological Association*
Trans. N.Y. Acad. Sci.	*Transactions of the New York Academy of Science*
Tr. Akad. Med. Nauk SSSR	*Trudy Akademiimeditsinskikh*
Tr. Inst. Fiziol. Im. I.P. Pavlov	*Trudy Instituta Fiziologicheskii Imeni I.P. Pavlov*
Tr. Inst. Vyss. Nerv. Dejat. Ser. Patofiziol.	*Trudy Instituta Vysshei Nervnoi Dejatel'nosti: Serii Fiziologicheskii*
Tr. Psikhiat. Klin. I.P. Pavlov	*Trudy Psikhiatrii Klinicheskoi I.P. Pavlov*
Univ. Calif. Chron.	*University of California Chronicle*
Univ. Calif. Publ. Psychol.	*University of California Publications in Psychology*
Univ. Iowa Stud. Child Welfare	*University of Iowa Studies in Child Welfare*
Vracheb. Delo	*Vrachebnoe delo Ministerstvo*
Wien. Arch. Psychol. Psychiat. Neurol.	*Wiener Archiv für Psychologie, Psychiatrie und Neurologie*
Yale J. Biol. Med.	*Yale Journal of Biology and Medicine*

Z. Biol.	*Zeitschrift für Biologie*
Z. Ges. Neurol. Psychiat.	*Zeitschrift für die gesamte Neurologie*
	und Psychiatrie
Z. Nevropat. Psikhiat.	*Zhurnal Nevropatologii i Psikhiatrii*
(Korsakoff)	*Imeni S. S. Korsakova*
Z. Psychosom. Med.	*Zeitschrift für psychosomatische Medizin*
Z. Vyss. Nerv. Dejat.	*Zhurnal Vysshei Nervnoi Dejatel' Nosti*
Pavlova	*Imeni I.P. Pavlova*

INDEX OF NAMES

SUBJECT INDEX

236